Nursing Skills in Supporting Mobility

T0002777

The ability to move easily and purposively contributes enormously to a sense of health and wellbeing, enabling increased independence and self-protection. However, many of the patients you encounter will have some degree of immobility whether it is temporary (for instance, due to local anaesthesia), permanent (for instance, due to amputation or stroke) or variable (for instance, due to arthritis or morbid obesity). This practical pocket guide covers:

- the anatomy and physiology of the musculoskeletal system
- the principles of ergonomics
- safe moving and handling practices
- positioning the patient
- performing a range of movement exercises
- legal aspects of moving and handling
- the promotion of sleep.

This competency-based text covers relevant key concepts, anatomy and physiology, lifespan matters, assessment and nursing skills. To support your learning, it also includes learning outcomes, concept map summaries, activities, questions and scenarios with sample answers and critical reflection thinking points.

Quick and easy to reference, this short, clinically-focused guide is ideal for use on placements or for revision. It is suitable for pre-registration nurses, students on the nursing associate programme and newly qualified nurses.

Sheila Cunningham is an Associate Professor in Adult Nursing at Middlesex University, UK. She has a breadth of experience teaching nurses both pre- and post-registration and she mentors clinicians supporting students in practice. She is also a Middlesex University Teaching Fellow and holds a Principal Fellowship at the Higher Education Academy. Her current role is Director for Learning, Teaching and Quality (School of Health and Education).

Tina Moore is a Senior Lecturer in Adult Nursing at Middlesex University, UK. She teaches nursing assessment, clinical skills and care interventions for both pre-qualifying and post-qualifying nurses. She is also a Middlesex University Teaching Fellow.

Skills in Nursing Practice

Series editors
Tina Moore, *Middlesex University, UK*
Sheila Cunningham, *Middlesex University, UK*

This series of competency-based pocket guides covers relevant key concepts, anatomy and physiology, lifespan matters, assessment and nursing skills for good clinical practice in a range of areas from safety and protection to promoting homeostasis. To support your learning, they include learning outcomes, concept map summaries, activities, questions and scenarios with sample answers and critical reflection thinking points.

Quick and easy to reference, these short, skills-focused texts are ideal for use on placements or for revision. They are ideal for pre-registration nurses, students on the nursing associate programme and newly qualified nurses feeling in need of a little revision.

List of Titles:

Nursing Skills in Professional and Practice Contexts
Tina Moore and Sheila Cunningham

Nursing Skills in Safety and Protection
Sheila Cunningham and Tina Moore

Nursing Skills in Nutrition, Hydration and Elimination
Sheila Cunningham and Tina Moore

Nursing Skills in Cardiorespiratory Assessment and Monitoring
Tina Moore and Sheila Cunningham

Nursing Skills in Supporting Mobility
Sheila Cunningham and Tina Moore

Nursing Skills in Control and Coordination
Tina Moore and Sheila Cunningham

For more information about this series, please visit: www.routledge.com/Skills-in-Nursing-Practice/book-series/SNP

Nursing Skills in Supporting Mobility

Sheila Cunningham and Tina Moore

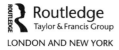

Routledge
Taylor & Francis Group

LONDON AND NEW YORK

First published 2021
by Routledge
2 Park Square, Milton Park, Abingdon, Oxon OX14 4RN

and by Routledge
605 Third Avenue, New York, NY 10158

Routledge is an imprint of the Taylor & Francis Group, an informa business

© 2021 Sheila Cunningham and Tina Moore

The right of **Sheila Cunningham and Tina Moore** to be identified as authors of this work has been asserted by them in accordance with sections 77 and 78 of the Copyright, Designs and Patents Act 1988.

British Library Cataloguing-in-Publication Data
A catalogue record for this book is available from the British Library

Library of Congress Cataloging-in-Publication Data
Names: Cunningham, Sheila, author. | Moore, Tina, author.
Title: Nursing skills in supporting mobility /
Sheila Cunningham and Tina Moore.
Description: Milton Park, Abingdon, Oxon; New York, NY: Routledge, 2021.
Series: Skills in nursing practice |
Includes bibliographical references and index. |
Summary: "The ability to move easily and purposively contributes enormously to a sense of health and wellbeing, enabling increased independence and self-protection. However, many of the patients you encounter will have some degree of immobility whether it is temporary (for instance, due to local anaesthesia), permanent (for instance, due to amputation or stroke) or variable (for instance, due to arthritis or morbid obesity). This concise guide covers: The anatomy and physiology of the musculoskeletal system The principles of ergonomics Safe moving and handling practices Positioning the patient Performing range of movement exercises Legal aspects of moving and handling The promotion of sleep. This competency-based text covers relevant key concepts, anatomy and physiology, lifespan matters, assessment, and nursing skills. To support your learning, it also includes learning outcomes, concept map summaries, activities, questions and scenarios with sample answers, and critical reflection thinking points. Quick and easy to reference, this short, clinically-focused guide is ideal for use on placements or for revision. It is suitable for pre-registration nurses, students on the nursing associate programme and newly qualified nurses"–Provided by publisher.
Identifiers: LCCN 2020044618 (print) | LCCN 2020044619 (ebook) |
ISBN 9781138479524 (hardback) | ISBN 9781138479555

ISBN: 978-1-138-47952-4 (hbk)
ISBN: 978-1-138-47955-5 (pbk)
ISBN: 978-1-351-06558-0 (ebk)

Typeset in Stone Serif
By Deanta Global Publishing Services, Chennai, India

Contents

Figures

FIGURES

Introduction to the *Skills in Nursing Practice* series

This particular book is one in a series of six *'Nursing Skills in...'* books.

Book 1 *Professional Skills and Practice Context*
Book 2 *Protection and Safety*
Book 3 *Acquisition of Nutrients and Removal of Waste*
Book 4 *Control and Co-ordination*
Book 5 *Cardiorespiratory Assessment and Monitoring*
Book 6 *Supporting Mobility*

These books are designed to be used in clinical practice and can be used not only for reference but also as an invaluable revision tool. There is a continuing emphasis on skills acquisition and development particularly within nursing. This is accompanied by the increasing understanding of the necessity to effectively and efficiently integrate theory and clinical skill competence-based learning. In doing so, these books hope to ensure that nurses have the best opportunity to become fit to practice and develop key employability skills. Therefore, each chapter has been linked to the *Future Nurse Proficiencies* (NMC 2018) which will enable you to map your skills development in relation to the standards set by the professional body.

The structure of each chapter within the books draws on constructivist pedagogical approaches and assimilation theory. Each chapter presents interlinking ideas and information through the use of concept maps. It is anticipated that the use of key words and connections will deepen and enhance those linkages from the concepts, drawing on the general and specific aspects of a topic, and will therefore promote active learning.

Concept maps are pictures or graphic representations that will help you to organise and represent your knowledge of a subject. This is achieved through helping you to link, differentiate and relate concepts to one another. They (concept maps) begin with a main idea (or concept) and then branch out to show how that main idea can be broken down into specific topics. They can also visually represent relationships between concepts and ideas in a quick, easy-to-understand format. Concept mapping is becoming increasingly popular as a means of teaching and learning within education. The introduction of concept maps will provide a quick summary with additional key information about the material in the *Clinical Skills for Nursing* book. We have also included related anatomy and physiology together with lifespan matters.

The end of each chapter will have questions (answers also provided) in the format of a quiz. This will help you to test your new knowledge, understanding and application of the content. There is also the opportunity for you to critically reflect on your learning using the SMART (Specific, Measurable, Achievable, Realistic and Time-bound) format. From this you should then be able to clearly identify areas for future development and learning.

These pocket-size books are not only designed to help develop your clinical skills (practice and knowledge) but also to improve your key transferrable skills, enabling them to advance your employability skills, i.e. problem solving; analytical and critical thinking; and team working. Therefore another aim for each book is to concentrate on scaffolding learning, therefore supporting, promoting and developing autonomous learning, questioning (informed) and critical thinking. The use of concept mapping allows the reorganisation of information in a visual manner to promote critical thinking in the nursing student. Through concept mapping students can see how ideas and patient care needs, and the interrelationships that exist between them, promote critical thinking in relation to clinical practice.

The books within this series are not designed to be comprehensive textbooks. They are the practice companions of the *Clinical Skills for Nursing Practice*, and are designed to be used in conjunction with that book. The design of these 'pocket-size' books will enable students/readers to use them as a resource whilst working within and outside of clinical practice.

Tina Moore and Sheila Cunningham

Introduction and overview

Protecting patients and ensuring safety is key to quality nursing care. The Nursing and Midwifery Council (2015) assert that nurses have a responsibility not only for the safety and protection of patients and the public but also for themselves. Evidence-based, best practice approaches are essential to enable meeting the needs of care and support with mobility and safety, accurately assessing the person's capacity for independence and self-care and initiating appropriate interventions. Understanding how movement and mobility develops and alters, together with being efficient and effective, is core to this. Good musculoskeletal (MSK) health is integral to an active and independent life, as well as enabling people with functional mobility issues (including balance, co-ordination and dexterity) to reach optimal mobility, in addition to contributing to muscular strength and endurance. This is essential to nearly all forms of work and life activities. Good MSK health also enhances physical and mental fitness and reduces the occurrence of other health problems.

Nurses also have a role in protecting themselves and thus use of proper procedures to enable people to move and mobilise is key to ensuring they are working safely and protecting their physical wellbeing. Musculoskeletal problems, especially lower back injuries, are still a significant problem among health care workers as well as the general population.

All employers have a legal responsibility to ensure the health and safety at work of their staff. Health and safety includes the prevention of accidents and work-related ill health, specifically musculoskeletal disorders (MSDs), back pain and upper limb disorders (ULDs). The Health and Safety at Work Act 1974 places general duties on employers and others. There are a number of other regulations which also add to this and impose specific requirements. These include: Management of Health and Safety at Work Regulations 1999, Workplace (Health, Safety and Welfare) Regulations 1992 and Manual Handling Operations Regulations 2002 Anyone working in a hospital, nursing home or community setting should not be in a position where they put their safety at risk such as lifting patients manually, which has been banned for some time. The use of equipment such as hoists, sliding aids and other specialised equipment means that staff should no longer have to risk injury while working. Patients can often do a lot for themselves and ought to be encouraged, or shown how, and this will also be of benefit to them. The key to this is awareness of anatomy and the physiology of movements, improving and encouraging independent mobility and support, ensuring risks are assessed and that resources are available and used correctly.

CHAPTER 1

Overview of musculoskeletal components and movement

Sheila Cunningham

Overview

The musculoskeletal system provides form, stability and movement to the human body. It consists of the body's bones (which make up the skeleton), muscles, tendons, ligaments, joints, cartilage and other connective tissue.

Link to *Future Nurse Proficiencies* (NMC 2018)

Platform 4 Providing and evaluating care (specifically, 4.7).

Annexe B: Nursing procedures, Section 7: Use evidence-based, best practice approaches for meeting needs for care and support with mobility and safety, accurately assessing the person's capacity for independence and self-care and initiating appropriate interventions.

Expected knowledge

- Connective tissue and general role of the musculoskeletal system
- Correct posture and consequences of poor posture.

Introduction

One of the four tissues types in the body is 'connective tissue'. This term describes the tissue that supports and binds tissues and organs together, namely ligaments and tendons. The chief components are collagen and elastic fibres, which are composed of a variety of different proteins. This enables them not only to be strong and durable but also flexible and elastic. In normal everyday activities, the range, speed and duration of movements cause stress on muscles, bones and connective tissues. These physical stresses and forces contribute to strength, resilience and endurance of the MSK but can also subject the system to over-stressing, causing trauma or degeneration. This may be seen in certain areas such as sport, in damage to ligaments or when a person falls and sprains an ankle. To really understand this a nurse ought to be aware of the structures, forces and processes which contribute to these movements, in addition to understanding the consequences if movements are incomplete, excessive or in some cases impossible due to other traumas or developmental problems. Whilst anatomy can be a challenging topic to grasp, it is a core element to understanding activities of daily living (walking/moving); it is the evidence that underpins assessment, decisions and care practices.

Content

Bones structure and function	Ossification	Types of body movements
Skeletal muscle structure and function	Posture and movement	Joints

Learning outcomes

- Outline the components of the musculoskeletal system
- Describe the process of bone growth, ossification and changes with age
- Differentiate the different joints and types of body movements and processes involved including lever systems
- Explain the terms and significance of biomechanics and ergogenics to movement.

Key background

Bone growth is dynamic and undergoes a continuous process termed 'modelling' and 'remodelling'. Through this older bone tissue is gradually replaced by new bone tissue in a continuous way. It is estimated that every bone in the body is completely reformed about every ten years (MSD, 2020); though this is conjecture, it reflects the dynamic process. All bones have essentially the same structure: a hard outer part (cortical bone) and a softer inner part (trabecular bone). This latter part is less dense than the hard outer part but still contributes significantly to bone strength. A reduction in the amount or quality of trabecular bone increases the risk of fractures (breaks). In order to maintain bone density and strength an adequate supply of calcium, vitamin D and other materials are necessary. Hormones also contribute to bone health: growth hormones, calcitonin, parathyroid hormones, oestrogen and testosterone. Weight-bearing activities (e.g. walking, jogging, skipping) where the limbs propel the body into a movement help bones strengthen by encouraging bone generation and remodelling. From this the softer inner bone (trabecular bone) develops into a complex lattice structure that confers a lightweight resistant structure and this strength decreases the probability of fractures and deformities occurring. Additionally, bones are covered by a thin membrane called the periosteum which is innervated and has a good blood supply important for growth. This is the reason fractures of bones are painful since bone tissue is not innervated, and thus pain signals are transmitted through periosteal innervation.

Rickets is a condition that was prevalent some years ago and not so much of late but still appears. It is a classic example of bone growth impacted by dietary problems. It affects bone development in children causing bone pain, poor growth and soft, weak bones that can lead to bone deformities. It has mostly disappeared in the western world after foods like cereal were fortified with vitamin D. A small increase in the incidence of cases of childhood rickets in the UK is reputed to be due to low levels of vitamin D in the blood. This is corrected by supplementing with vitamin D which shows the range of knowledge required in all areas of nursing such as assessment of childhood growth and development, nutritional adequacy and advice for maintaining it. This is not unique to children and occurs in adults too; however, it is then termed 'osteomalacia' or 'osteopenia'.

Nurses have a professional responsibility to maintain the knowledge and skills needed for safe and effective practice and to recognise and work within the limits of their competence (NMC, 2018). This also refers to the fundamental knowledge of human functioning which is widely taught within nursing undergraduate programmes and applied regularly within the practice setting. The issue with MSK is that it also applies to nurses' own physical health and wellbeing not just that of their patients.

MUSCULOSKELETAL SYSTEM

BONES perform five main functions for the body:

- **Provide support**: structural framework and attachment of soft tissues and organs.
- **Store minerals and lipids**: Calcium (93%) and phosphates. Energy reserves as lipids (fats – as yellow marrow).
- **Produce blood cells**: Red and white blood cells, other blood elements (red marrow).
- **Protect body organs**: e.g. rib cage protects heart and lungs, skull protects the brain, vertebrae protect the spinal cord.
- **Provide leverage and movement**: can change the magnitude (strength) and direction of the forces generated by muscles.

The **musculoskeletal system** are TWO systems which function together in an integrated way.
It provides form, support, stability, and movement to the body.
Consists of *bones of the skeleton, muscles, cartilage, tendons, ligaments, joints,* and other connective tissue that supports and binds tissues and organs together.

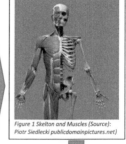

Figure 1 Skelton and Muscles (Source): Piotr Siedlecki publicdomainpictures.net)

FRAMEWORK – *joined up (connective tissue)*
Ligaments: connect bone to bone, **Tendons:** connect muscle to bone.

TWO key CELLS: **OSTEOBLAST** (formation) & **OSTEOCLAST** (resorption)

Bone strength and thickness relate to stresses:
- Heavy activity = osteoblast formation and density
- Reduced activity = increased osteoclast or loss of density

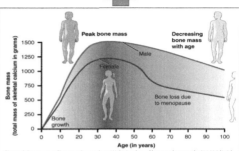

Figure 2 Bone mass (Source: Connexions Web site. http://cnx.org/content/col11496/1.6/, Jun 19, 2013. / CC BY (https://creativecommons.org/licenses/by/3.0)

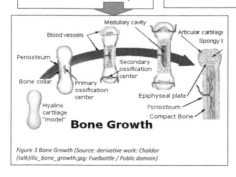

Figure 3 Bone Growth (Source: derivative work: Chaldor (talk)Illu_bone_growth.jpg: Fuelbottle / Public domain)

Skeletal structure
Consists of **208 bones**
Specialised connective tissue (collagen matrix, calcium phosphate and carbonate)
Bone formation and breakdown (*resorption*) occur continuously:
- Formation exceed resorption in children (*increase/growth*)
- Formation and resorption balance in adulthood (*static*)
- Resorption exceed formation in old age (*decrease*)

FIGURE 1.1 Musculoskeletal system

Development of the spinal curves

Children's spines naturally curve in stages:

- Foetal development: primary curves in the thoracic spine develop, as well as the sacral curve at the bottom of the spine.
- Babies: C-shaped spine.
- Infant: secondary curves in the cervical and lumbar spine develop as infants become able to lift their heads, sit up, crawl, stand, and walk.
- Adolescent/adult: spine continues to develop natural curves into a normal, mature spine with curves (two convex and two concave).

Maintaining spinal curves: considerations

- Babies/toddlers: good posture unless abnormality. All four curves in alignment.
- Tall children tend to droop their shoulders. Carrying heavy bags causes shortening of fascia and neck muscles.
- Adults: sedentary work/life effects curves of the spine. Strong abdominal muscles.
- Elderly: not automatically a problem but poor posture, gravity, use of aids for movement – all contribute to 'stoop' posture.

The sections of the spine have specific names.

- The **cervical** spine refers to the neck.
- The **thoracic** spine refers to the chest.
- The **lumbar** spine and sacral spine refer to the lower back.

POSTURE AND SPINE DEVELOPMENT

Purposive movement the body must move in a synchronised manner.
Movements ought to be smooth and coordinated with appropriate force for the intended movement/task.

Posture – key is spine.
Bones (vertebrae) joined by muscles and ligaments.
Flat, soft discs separate and cushion the vertebrae from each other.
The spine is thus flexible for movements.

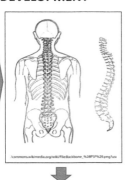

/commons.wikimedia.org/wiki/File:Backbone_%28PSF%29.png?us

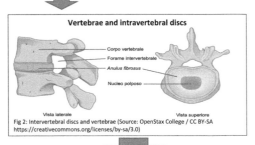

Vertebrae and intravertebral discs

Corpo vertebrale
Forame intervertebrale
Anulus fibrosus
Nucleo polposo

Vista laterale   Vista superiore
Fig 2: Intervertebral discs and vertebrae (Source: OpenStax College / CC BY-SA https://creativecommons.org/licenses/by-sa/3.0)

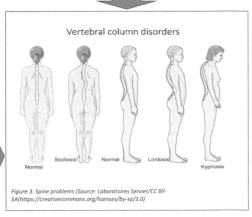

Vertebral column disorders

Scoliosis   Normal   Lordosis
Normal   Kyphosis

Figure 3. Spine problems (Source: Laboratoires Servier/CC BY-SA(https://creativecommons.org/licenses/by-sa/3.0)

FIGURE 1.2 Posture and spine development

JOINTS AND MOVEMENT

Tendons and ligaments

Tendons and ligaments are fibrous bands of connective tissue. Both stabilise the skeleton and allow movement. Both contain Collagen – ligaments more elastic than tendons. Several factors can increase the risk of injury, including:

- overuse, e.g. through playing sports, trauma from a fall or blow.
- twisting the tendon or ligament into an awkward position.
- weakness in the surrounding muscles due to a sedentary lifestyle.

Strain – trauma from falling or suddenly twisting especially those who are inactive.
Sprain – ligament stretches and tears.
Treatment: RICE
Rest the injured area and no weight on it.
Ice the injury to reduce swelling and pain.
Compression **(bandage)** to reduce swelling.
Elevate above the heart level (eases pain and swelling). May also add non-steroidal anti-inflammatory drugs.

Conditions affecting the joints

Arthritis is an inflammatory condition of a synovial joint.

- **Osteoarthritis**, in which the cartilage is damaged over time and thins until pressure between the bones causes pain. Effects hands, knees, hips and spine.
- **Rheumatoid arthritis** is an autoimmune condition in which the immune system attacks the tissues of the joints, causing damage.

Gout occurs when uric acid crystals build up in a synovial joint (usually the big toe), causing pain. May also inflame due to overuse termed **Synovitis. Symptoms:** pain, tenderness, stiffness, inflammation.

Figure 1 Synovial joint (Source: OpenStax College / CC BY (https://creativecommons.org/licenses/by/3.0))

Walking – muscles

Several each acting at a different joint at a different phase e.g.
Gluteus maximus –hip to decelerate the forward motion of the lower limb.
Quadriceps femoris – keeps the leg extended at knee.
Anterior compartment of the leg – maintains the ankle dorsiflexion, positioning the heel for the strike.
Hamstring muscles – extend the hip.
Iliopsoas and rectus femoris – flex the thigh.
TERMS:
Trendelenburg gait: leaning on affected side (weak gluteals)
Apraxia/Dyspraxia – poor coordinated movements
Bradykinesia – unusually slow movements

WALKING – *gait PUTTING IT ALL TOGETHER*

Coordinated process – a tactic called the **double pendulum**.

- During forward motion, the leg that leaves the ground swings forward from the hip (first pendulum).
- Foot then strikes the ground with the heel of the foot and rolls through to the toe in a motion (inverted pendulum).
- The motion is coordinated so that one foot or the other is always in contact with the ground.
Repeated cycle ....

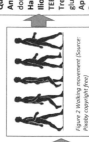

Figure 2 Walking movement (Source: Pixaby copyright free)

FIGURE 1.3 Joints and movement

MUSCLES AND LEVERS TO MOVE THE HUMAN BODY

MUSCLES
There are 3 key muscle tissue types only one of which is involved in body movement.

Skeletal muscle – voluntary movement

Cardiac muscle – heart contractions

Smooth muscle – involuntary organ movements (e.g. digestive tract)

SKELETAL MUSCLE – Bundles – Striped (striated). **Structures**

Sarcomeres shorten (slide together) = *muscle shorten = bones move*

LEVERS and MOVEMENT

There are four parts to a lever – **lever arm, pivot, effort and load** and three classes of levers

- bones act as *lever arms*
- joints act as *pivots*
- muscles provide the *effort forces* to move loads
- load forces are body parts that are moved or forces needed to lift, push or pull things outside our bodies.

Class 3: Bending the forearm

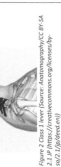

Figure 4 Class 3 lever (Source: OpenStax / CC BY (https://creativecommons.org/licenses/by/4.0)

LOAD

EFFORT

PIVOT

Movement

Class 1: Lever holding the head up

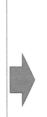

EFFORT

LOAD

PIVOT

Figure 2 Class 1 lever (Source: Anatomography/CC BY-SA 2.1 JP (https://creativecommons.org/licenses/by-sa/2.1/jp/deed.en)

Class 2: Standing on tiptoes

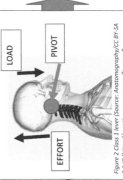

EFFORT

LOAD

PIVOT

Figure 3 Class 2 lever (Source: / CC BY (https://creativecommons.org/licenses/by/4.0)

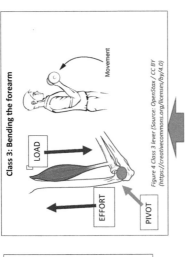

Figure 1 Muscle composition (Source: Creative Commons Attribution-ShareAlike 3.0)

FIGURE 1.4 Muscles and levers to move the human body

TYPES OF BODY MOVEMENTS

TERMINOLOGY:
Muscles – enable movements – **TYPES** of movement include:

Flexion. The state of being bent. The cervical spine is flexed when the chin is moved toward the chest.

Extension. The state of being in a straight line. The cervical spine is extended when the head is held straight.

Hyperextension. The state of exaggerated extension. The cervical spine is hyperextended when the person looks overhead, toward the ceiling.

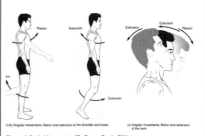

Figure 1 Body Movements (By Tonye Ogele CNX - http://cnx.org/content/m46398/latest/?collection=col11496/latest, CC BY-SA 3.0, https://commons.wikimedia.org/w/index.php?curid=63388586)

Abduction. Lateral movement of a body part away from the midline of the body. The arm is abducted when it is held away from the body.

Adduction. Lateral movement of a body part toward the midline of the body. The arm is adducted when it is moved from an outstretched position toward the body.

Rotation. Turning of a body part around an axis. The head is rotated (around the cervical spine) when moved from side to side to indicate "no."

Circumduction. Rotating an extremity in a complete circle. Circumduction is a combination of abduction, adduction, extension, and flexion.

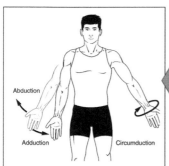

Figure 2 More Body Movements (By Tonye Ogele CNX - http://cnx.org/content/m46398/latest/?collection=col11496/latest, CC BY-SA 3.0, https://commons.wikimedia.org/w/index.php?curid=63388586)

Supination. The palm or sole is rotated in an upward position

Pronation. The palm of the hand or sole of the foot is rotated in a downward position.

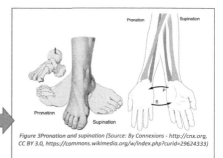

Figure 3 Pronation and supination (Source: By Connexions - http://cnx.org, CC BY 3.0, https://commons.wikimedia.org/w/index.php?curid=29624333)

FIGURE 1.5 Types of body movements

ERGONOMICS AND BIOMECHANICS IN MOVEMENT

Ergonomics and body movements

- Ergonomics is the study of the relationship between workers and designs of their working environments.
- Tasks, equipment, information and the environment suit each worker.
- In healthcare settings, employers are required to provide equipment to help nurses to maintain good posture when undertaking care activities.

Children and ergonomics

Children spend hours a day playing video/computer games and working on school projects.

Mismatch between a child's body size and the size of adult furniture and computer equipment.

Challenges presented by children:

- Range of body sizes
- Rate of growth (obesity)
- Strength capabilities (muscle fibres)
- Cognitive characteristics (biomechanics/action for various activities)

Children – ergonomic risks

- School backpacks (too heavy, no more than 15% body weight) though the link to back pain in children is controversial (Yamato et al., 2018).
- Poor posture (slouching, reclining).
- Age appropriate furniture (chair/desk/computer) and position.
- Lighting and 'computer vision' aspects.

Balance – the ability to maintain the line of gravity.

Age, gender, and height have all been shown to impact an individual's ability to balance.

Biomechanics and body movements

- Related to ergonomics and complement each other in promoting healthy back and natural postures.
- The 'application of physical laws of mechanics' to understand the human body movements. (Newton's Laws of Motion)
- Relationship between external forces and structures of bones, joints, muscles and ligaments (Polak, 2011).
- Based on the use of the body's centre of gravity, stable leg base for balance, keeping the head up and bending the knees slightly, to maintain natural the spinal curves – use natural LEVERS to move objects or self
- Force from lifting heavy loads or poor postures is pain, intervertebral disc degeneration and collapse.

Recommended position for sitting at a computer

1. Sit well back in the seat, ensure back is supported with backrest.
2. Adjust height of the chair to ensure forearms are horizontal when using the keyboard.
3. Wrists in neutral position or L shape when using keyboard.
4. Feet flat on the floor or use a foot rest so knees equal or lower than hips.
5. Check height and angle of screen to hold head in a comfortable position (5cm above eyeline).
6. Documents or other items within easy reach.
7. Take frequent breaks to move (NHS, 2019).

Ergonomics Checklist – sitting at a computer

- Shoulders should be relaxed
- Forearms & hands in a straight line (90 degrees)
- Thigh should be horizontal to floor.
- Chair should provide lower back support
- Feet should be flat on floor
- Top of screen should be at or slightly below eye level (15 to 30 degrees below line of sight)
- Monitor should be arms-length away from face. (18" to 24" away from screen)
- Position screen to avoid reflected glare

Figure 1 Sitting at a computer (Source: Brown educ 491 at English Wikibooks/Public domain)

FIGURE 1.6 Ergonomics and biomechanics

Activity: now test yourself

1. Bone is constantly being made and remodelled. What two cells are involved in this process? Choose **two**.

   a) osteocytes

   b) osteoblasts

   c) chondrocytes

   d) chondyle

   e) osteoclasts

   f) osteomalacia.

2. There are three classes of levers (load, pivot and force) which create movement. If a person is standing up on their tiptoes to reach an object, what type of lever is this? What are the elements of this lever?

3. Define these terms:

a) abduction	
b) extension	
c) pronation	
d) flexion	
e) rotation	
f) biomechanics	

4. How many curves are there in the human adult spine?

   a) three

   b) four

   c) five

d) six

e) two.

5. How many curves are there in an infant spine?

a) three

b) four

c) five

d) six

e) two.

6. What does the term 'lordosis' refer to?

a) the inward curve of the lumbar spine (just above the buttocks/gluteals) and the slightly extended gluteal area

b) the arched structure of the thoracic spine (hunchback)

c) the outer curve of the lumbar spine in a hunched over position

d) the curvature of the cervical spine and rounded shoulders.

Answers

1. b) and e). *Osteoblasts are immature bone-producing cells – when the bone is mature these become osteocytes. Osteoclasts are the resorption or remodellers and terms which commence with 'chondro' refer to cartilage, the early stage of bone development which is overtaken by the osteoblasts.*

2. This is an example of the **second** class lever. The **load** is the weight of the body being lifted. The **pivot** is between the metatarsals and phalanges (toes). The **force** is the gastrocnemius muscles as it contracts to pull the heel upwards. *This is a common feature in sport training or developing activity and muscle strength exercises for walking.*

3. Definitions:

a) abduction	Lateral movement of a body part away from the midline of the body. The arm is abducted when it is held away from the body.
b) extension	The state of being in a straight line. The cervical spine is extended when the head is held straight.
c) pronation	When the palm of the hand or sole of the foot is rotated in a downward position.
d) flexion	The state of being bent. The cervical spine is flexed when the chin is moved toward the chest.
e) rotation	The turning of a body part around an axis. The head is rotated (around the cervical spine) when moved from side to side to indicate 'no'.
f) biomechanics	The 'application of physical laws of mechanics' to understand the human body movements. The relationship between external forces and structures of bones, joints, muscles and ligaments to move objects or the body itself. Related to ergonomics.

4. b) four. *There are two concave and two convex which give the unique 'S' shape curve structure of the adult spine from the neck to the coccyx.*

5. e) two. *On first being born a child has one to reflect the 'C' shape; as the infant sits up and gains control of their head, the curves begin to develop and this is then described as* **two** *curves.*

6. a). *This curvy feature, the lower part of the 'S' spine shape where the gluteals look to be protruding out a little, is quite normal – it can be an excessive curve of the lower back and lead to excess pressure on the spine, causing pain and discomfort.*

Reflection: ask yourself

1. What do I know now that I didn't know before?

2. What am I confused/unclear about?

3. What areas do I need to focus on?

4. My action plan for further learning (make objectives SMART – Specific/Measurable/Achievable/Realistic/Time-bound):

CHAPTER 2

Movement assessment and exercises

Sheila Cunningham

Overview

The musculoskeletal (MSK) system enables movement which is mainly voluntary and purposeful. However there are limits to the types and ranges of movements which can cause damage to or result from problems with the musculoskeletal system.

Link to *Future Nurse Proficiencies* (NMC 2018)

Platform 4 Providing and evaluating care (specifically, 4.7).

Annexe B: Nursing procedures, Section 7: Use evidence-based, best practice approaches for meeting needs for care and support with mobility and safety, accurately assessing the person's capacity for independence and self-care and initiating appropriate interventions.

Expected knowledge

- Body movement and gait
- Inflammation and general degeneration processes.

Introduction

Nurses need good assessment skills to care for all patients but in the case of people with MSK problems, nurses need to be especially alert to the often chronic and debilitating nature of the conditions and consequent problems which this brings. This requires a holistic approach to assessment, aiming to enable patients to be as independent as possible. Some inflammatory conditions of MSK can affect any age group, young or old, and impact on movement and activities of daily living. MSK conditions is a broad term, encompassing approximately 200 different conditions that affect the muscles, joints and skeleton. Approximately ten million adults, and around 12,000 children, have a MSK condition in England (DH, 2019). Many major MSK conditions can be avoided, or their symptoms reduced, by staying active throughout the life course, ensuring there is a range of balance and strength activities, a healthy diet and protection and support in the workplace. Public Health England (PHE) launched the Musculoskeletal Health Improvement programme in April 2018. This was a result of the need to act on the Global Burden of Disease (GBD) data, which requires a whole-system public health approach to MSK health (PHE, 2019).

Content

Assessment of mobility	Movement and exercise	Immobility and consequences
Range of motion assessments	Assessment tools	Promoting independence

Learning outcomes

- Outline the assessment process and associated tools which may be used
- Rationalise the use of active versus passive exercises for strength development
- Explain the consequences of immobility to the health of individuals
- Describe a range of exercises people who are immobilised in bed may be encouraged to do.

Key background

Musculoskeletal (MSK)-related pain has a major impact on individuals and society with back, neck, shoulder and knee pain being the most commonly reported MSK problems (WHO, 2021). MSK-related pain is the second most common reason for general practitioner (GP) visits. It also accounts for approximately 20–30% of all GP consultations in the UK. MSK problems and related resulting conditions such as mental health problems are responsible for a substantial amount of poor health, and place a substantial burden on the NHS and other care services. Low back and neck pain has a severe impact on quality of life, resulting in disability with chronic joint pain or osteoarthritis affecting over 8.75 million people in the UK (DH, 2019). In the workplace, almost 30 million working days are lost due to MSK conditions every year in the UK, which account for almost 20% of all reported sickness conditions (ONS, 2018). This is however an improvement on the 2016 data of 22.4% (ONS, 2016). As the population ages, there are more people potentially living with MSK conditions, and together with changes to retirement age this may mean that people need to work longer with an MSK condition. Additionally, there are wide inequalities in the prevalence of long-term MSK conditions. Women are reported to be more affected than men; also some ethnicities (such as Irish) report more issues than others. There are also links to deprivation and low income (PHE, 2019).

In their longer-term plan, the NHS prioritises MSK conditions including degenerative conditions such as arthritis and injuries such as back pain, advocating expanding access to support beyond general practitioners, for example the online ESCAPE pain (Enabling Self-management and Coping with Arthritic Pain through Exercise) programme. This emphasises the need for society and nurses working in every field of care to be aware of movement processes, causes and consequences of MSK degeneration or injury and to be able to assess and plan care appropriately.

Nurses have a professional responsibility to maintain the knowledge and skills required for safe and effective practice and to recognise and work within the limits of their competence (NMC, 2018). Clients/patients with MSK-related conditions are an example of a group who will be cared for within the wider allied health profession services (physiotherapists, occupational therapists, diagnostic radiographers, dietitians, orthoptists, osteopaths, podiatrists, prosthetists/orthotists, therapeutic radiographers). This highlights the team approach to care and contribution of many professionals and thus the knowledge required of what each professional contributes and how they can seamlessly connect with each other towards patient care.

ASSESSMENT OF MOBILITY

Nursing assessment:

Aim: to establish the patient's ability to mobilise and independence and to determine the level of assistance required to address their activities of daily living. To observe and dashes ability to manage walking, using stairs/steps and any risks to personal safety and mobility. Ask:

- Is the patient able to stand, walk, and go to the toilet?
- Is the patient able to move up and down, roll and turn in bed?
- Does the patient need equipment to mobilise?
- What is the level of power in their arms and legs?
- Does the patient have any history of falling?
- *If necessary – complete a separate Manual Handling Risk Assessment.*

Mobility assessment tools

- Barthel Index (BI) – measure of functional ability for a person to care for him/herself
- Direct observation or Self Report
- Ordinal scale: 0=unable, 1=needs help, 2=independent
- Newer version uses other numerical measures but instrument relates to the degree of independence
- Ability to perform 10 selfcare activities:
  - ○ Feeding
  - ○ Bathing
  - ○ Grooming
  - ○ Dressing
  - ○ Bowels
  - ○ Bladder
  - ○ Toilet use
  - ○ Transfer (bed to chair)
  - ○ Mobility (flat)
  - ○ Stairs

Mobility and predicting risk of falls (in elderly) Timed Up & Go test and Turn 180° (NICE, 2019)

Ensure the person is safe and confident to do this unaided. Do not do this if the person feels weak or unwell.

- Time the person getting up from a chair without using their arms, walking 3 metres, turning around, returning to the chair, and sitting down. If the person usually uses a walking aid, this can be used during the test.
- During the test, observe the person's postural stability, gait, stride length, and sway. Standardized cut-off scores to predict risk of falling have not yet been established. However, a score of 12–15 seconds or more may indicate high risk of falls in older people.
- Also consider: age of the person, the type of footwear, the use of a walking aid, and the general health of the person (American College of Rheumatology, 2015).
- Turn 180° test – Ask the person to stand up and step around until they are facing the opposite direction. If the person takes more than four steps, further assessment should be considered.

Oxford scale (ordinal 0–5 on muscle (often performed by Physiotherapist)

- **0/5** No contraction
- **1/5** Visible/palpable muscle contraction but no movement
- **2/5** Movement with gravity eliminated
- **3/5** Movement against gravity only
- **4/5** Movement against gravity with some resistance
- **5/5** Movement against gravity with full resistance

FIGURE 2.1 Assessment of mobility

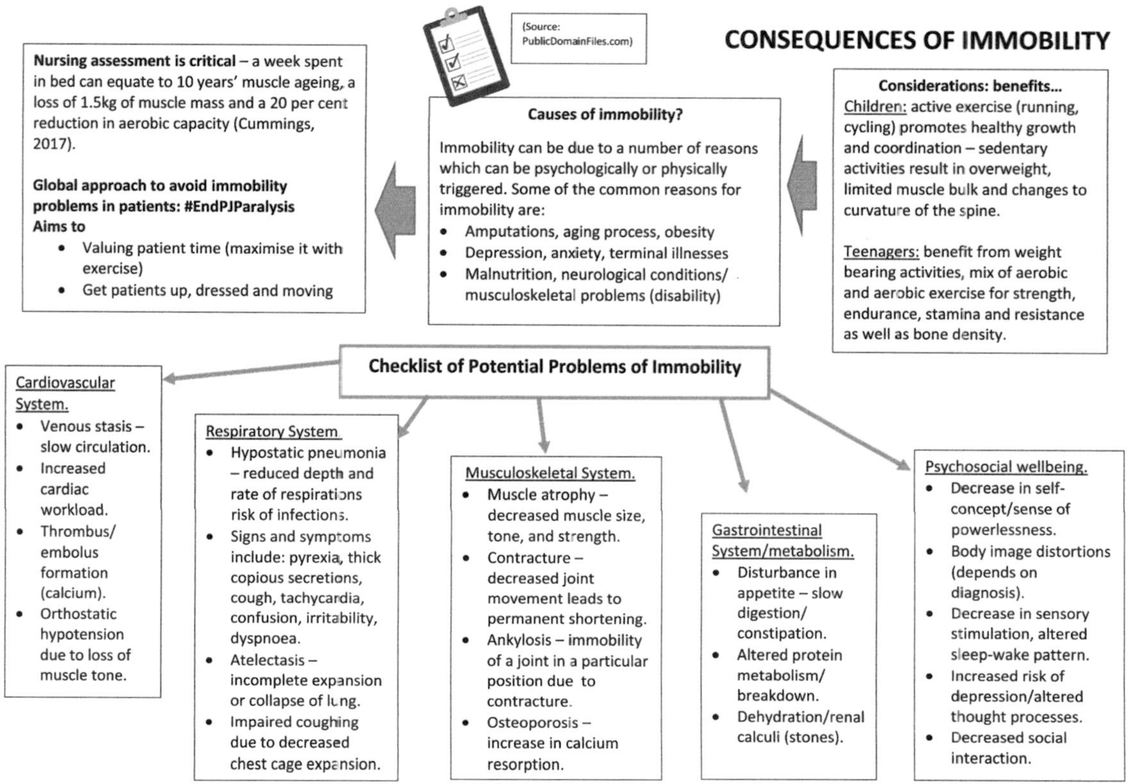

CONSEQUENCES OF IMMOBILITY

[Source: PublicDomainFiles.com]

Considerations: benefits...

Children: active exercise (running, cycling) promotes healthy growth and coordination – sedentary activities result in overweight, limited muscle bulk and changes to curvature of the spine.

Teenagers: benefit from weight bearing activities, mix of aerobic and aerobic exercise for strength, endurance, stamina and resistance as well as bone density.

Nursing assessment is critical – a week spent in bed can equate to 10 years' muscle ageing, a loss of 1.5kg of muscle mass and a 20 per cent reduction in aerobic capacity (Cummings, 2017).

Global approach to avoid immobility problems in patients: #EndPJParalysis
Aims to

- Valuing patient time (maximise it with exercise)
- Get patients up, dressed and moving

Causes of immobility?

Immobility can be due to a number of reasons which can be psychologically or physically triggered. Some of the common reasons for immobility are:

- Amputations, aging process, obesity
- Depression, anxiety, terminal illnesses
- Malnutrition, neurological conditions/ musculoskeletal problems (disability)

Checklist of Potential Problems of Immobility

Cardiovascular System.
- Venous stasis – slow circulation.
- Increased cardiac workload.
- Thrombus/ embolus formation (calcium).
- Orthostatic hypotension due to loss of muscle tone.

Respiratory System.
- Hypostatic pneumonia – reduced depth and rate of respirations risk of infections.
- Signs and symptoms include: pyrexia, thick copious secretions, cough, tachycardia, confusion, irritability, dyspnoea.
- Atelectasis – incomplete expansion or collapse of lung.
- Impaired coughing due to decreased chest cage expansion.

Musculoskeletal System.
- Muscle atrophy – decreased muscle size, tone, and strength.
- Contracture – decreased joint movement leads to permanent shortening.
- Ankylosis – immobility of a joint in a particular position due to contracture.
- Osteoporosis – increase in calcium resorption.

Gastrointestinal System/metabolism.
- Disturbance in appetite – slow digestion/ constipation.
- Altered protein metabolism/ breakdown.
- Dehydration/renal calculi (stones).

Psychosocial wellbeing.
- Decrease in self-concept/sense of powerlessness.
- Body image distortions (depends on diagnosis).
- Decrease in sensory stimulation, altered sleep-wake pattern.
- Increased risk of depression/altered thought processes.
- Decreased social interaction.

FIGURE 2.2 Consequences of immobility

ASSESSING RANGE OF MOTION

Upper extremities: Body part	Assessment	ROM
Neck	Patient bends head forward, backward ('nods') bends neck side to side.	Flexion/extension
	Turns head to look over their shoulder.	Rotation
Shoulder	Standing or sitting, the patient raises their arms to the vertical position (towards the ceiling). Then they bring arms down:	Flexion
	• Make small circular movements with arms at the sides.	Circumduction
	• Touches the opposite shoulder (across the body).	Adduction
	• Both hand clasp behind the neck.	External rotation/abduction
	• Then both hands reach back to the lower back.	Rotation
Elbow	Bend and straighten elbows.	Flexion/extension
	Arms hold onto the waist at the sides with elbows outwards.	Rotation
Wrist	Bend and straighten the wrist. Turn palm upward then downward.	Flexion/extension Pronation/supination
Hand	Make a fist and open it. Spread fingers out wider (stretch) then bring back together.	Flexion/extension Adduction/abduction

Lower extremities: Body Part	Assessment	ROM
Hips	Patient lies supine:	
	Straight leg, raise leg towards the ceiling then relax back.	Flexion
	Cross one leg over the other.	Abduction
	Swing legs laterally (right and left).	Adduction
Knees	Patient sits. Ask them to raise one foot keeping the knee in the sitting flexed position (extend from below the knee)	Extension
Ankles	With the foot held off the floor, patient points toes downwards and brings them back up	Plantar flexion Dorsiflexion
Toes	Turn sole of foot inwards and then outwards. Bend toes down and back.	Inversion/eversion Flexion/hyperextension

FIGURE 2.3 Assessment of range of motion

Types of exercises
- *Passive* – exercises are carried out by the nurse, without assistance from the patient. Will not preserve muscle mass or bone mineralisation because there is no voluntary contraction.
- *Active* – exercises performed by the patient themselves without assistance, to increase muscle strength. May also have some nurse assistance (*active assistive*).
- *Resistive* – active exercises performed by the patient by pulling or pushing against an opposing force.
- *Isometric* – exercises are performed by the patient by contracting and relaxing muscles (no shortening of muscle or moving a bone) e.g. pushing against a wall/solid object.

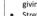

Figure 1 Active lower back exercises
(Source: Creative Commons license 3.0)

PASSIVE EXERCISES

THE PURPOSES OF EXERCISE FOR THE IMMOBILE PATIENT to...
- Maintain joint mobility – putting each of the patient's joints through all possible movements to increase and/or maintain movement in each joint.
- Prevent contracture, atony (insufficient muscular tone), and atrophy of muscles.
- Stimulate circulation,
- Improve coordination.
- Increase tolerance for more activity.
- Maintain and build muscle strength.

End of exercise period:
- Use passive exercises as required, however, encourage active exercises when the patient is able to do so.
- Evaluate the patient for fatigue, joint discomfort, and joint mobility.
- Document – ROM is often placed on a flow sheet or the nursing notes.
- If there is any adverse response to the exercises do note this. Ideally documents will indicate extent to which joints can be moved.
- If unsure ask the Physiotherapist for guidance and support – do work under the scope of practice.

Range of Motion (ROM) exercises – *procedure*
Carried out by physiotherapists and at times nurses.
- Plan when ROM exercises will be done. Gain patient consent and cooperation.
- Assess if the patient can do this themselves.
- Expect heart rate and respiratory rate to increase.

Frequency
- ROM exercise done at least twice a day.
- Bath is one appropriate time/location or before bedtime. Warm water relaxes the muscles and decreases spasticity of the joints
- Immobile patients exercise every eight hours to prevent contractures occurring.

Commencing ROM exercises
- Joints are exercised sequentially, from the neck moving downwards.
- Put each joint through the ROM procedure a minimum of three to five times (*see concept map ROM*).
- Avoid overexerting the patient; observe for this ROM movements slowly and gradually using smooth and rhythmic movements appropriate for the patient's condition.

During ROM exercise
- Support the joints of the limb extremity when giving passive exercise.
- Stretch the muscles and keep the joint flexible.
- Move each joint until there is resistance, but not pain.
- Keep friction at a minimum to avoid injuring the skin.
- Return the joint to its neutral position.

FIGURE 2.4 Passive exercises

EXERCISE FOR THOSE IMMOBILISED IN BED

Prolonged period in bed

This can occur due to a number of reasons and the key is to maintain muscle strength and tone as well as circulation. In addition exercises are encouraged to be done 'actively' by the patient or client and will contribute to wellbeing and recovery speed.
All other precautions against complications of bedrest ought to also be considered too.

A physiotherapist will usually advise exercises to be undertaken every hour if possible, with several repetitions e.g. 10 and for a set period such as 30 seconds, and also within energy and comfort ability. No warm up is required and it is recommended to perform a range of upper and lower body exercises.

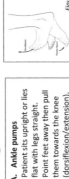

Figure 1

Dorsiflexion [Source: Connexions / CC BY (https://creativecommons. org/licenses/by/3.0)

A. Ankle pumps
1. Patient sits upright or lies flat with legs straight.
2. Point feet away then pull them towards the knee (dorsiflexion/extension).

B. Static quadricep contractions
1. Patient sits upright or lies flat with legs straight.
2. Pulls foot up (dorsiflexion) so that toes are pointing towards the ceiling.
3. Push the back of the knee down into the bed and tighten the muscle on the front of your thigh. Hold for 5 seconds, relax and repeat on each leg.

C. Gluteal squeeze
1. Patient asked to squeeze their buttock muscles together as tightly as possible.
2. Hold for a count of 5 seconds then relax for 10 seconds and repeat 10 times.

D. Heel slides
1. Patient sits upright or lies flat with legs straight.
2. Asked to bend one knee by sliding the heel up towards the bottom.
3. Then slowly straighten the same leg back out by sliding the heel away from the body
4. Repeat steps 10 times on each leg.

E. Arms push-ups
1. Patient lies on their back.
2. Asked to keep shoulders on bed raise arms inform to touch shoulders with the back of your hands (surrender position).
3. Then push arms up towards the ceiling and then return to the starting position. Repeat.

F. Shoulder raise
1. Patient starts with arms by their sides.
2. Lift your arms up above your head as far as you can.
3. Then slowly lower them back down.
4. Repeat steps 10 times.

End of exercise period:
- Use passive exercises as required, however, encourage active exercises when the patient is able to do so.
- Evaluate the patient for fatigue, joint discomfort, and joint mobility.
- Document – ROM is often placed on a flow sheet or the nursing notes.
- If there is any adverse response to the exercises do note this. Ideally documents will indicate extent to which joints can be moved.
- If unsure ask the Physiotherapist for guidance and support – do work under the scope of practice.

FIGURE 2.5 Exercises for those immobilised in bed

Activity: now test yourself

1. What is the difference between active and passive exercises?

2. What is the purpose of passive exercises for immobilised patients? A list will suffice.

3. What is the aim of assessing a patient's range of movement (ROM)?

   a) to determine the strength of the movement

   b) to explore the types of movements preferred

   c) to determine if the range of movement is within the expected range

   d) to determine if the movement is painful or not.

4. Give two examples of exercises recommended for people immobilised in bed.

Answers

1. **Passive exercises** are carried out by the nurse, without assistance from the patient. Will not preserve muscle mass or bone mineralisation because there is no voluntary contraction. **Active exercises** are performed by the patient themselves without assistance, to increase muscle strength. May also have some nurse assistance (active assistive).

2. The purpose of passive exercises is to:
   - *maintain joint mobility*
   - *prevent contracture, atony (insufficient muscular tone) and atrophy of muscles*
   - *stimulate circulation*
   - *improve coordination*
   - *increase tolerance for more activity*
   - *maintain and build muscle strength.*

3. c)

   If the movement is within the expected range this is positive. If not then exercises can enable development of this. If movements are painful then ROM assessment will not address this and may even limit ability to exercise and point to another problem which might need investigating.

4. Any of these:
   - *ankle-pumps (flexion and extension of the ankle and foot)*
   - *static quadricep contractions (leg staying flat on the bed and knee pushed down into the bed)*
   - *gluteal squeeze (tighten buttock muscles and clench)*
   - *heel-slides (legs lengthen along the bed and knees raised with heel sliding up towards buttocks then straightened again)*
   - *arm push-ups (supine position, arms pushing up towards the ceiling)*
   - *shoulder-raises (lift arms above the head).*

Reflection: ask yourself

1. What do I know now that I didn't know before?

2. What am I confused/unclear about?

3. What areas do I need to focus on?

4. My action plan for further learning (make objectives SMART – Specific/Measurable/Achievable/Realistic/Time-bound):

CHAPTER 3

Safe moving and handling practices

Tina Moore

Overview

Today, there should be no situation where nurses find themselves having to routinely manually lift patients. There are many safe alternatives for lifting (hoists, slide sheets, etc.). Patient care plans should now contain information about their mobility status (RCN, 2019) and a manual moving and handling risk assessment should be carried out.

Link to *Future Nurse Proficiencies* (NMC 2018)

Platform 3 Assessing needs and planning care (Section 3.2).
Platform 4 Prioritising and evaluating care (Section 4.12).
Annexe B, Part 1: Procedures for assessing people's needs for person-centred care. Specifically, 2.17: undertake a whole body systems assessment including respiratory, circulatory, neurological, musculoskeletal, cardiovascular and skin status.
Annexe B, Part 2: Procedures for the planning, provision and management of person-centred nursing care. Specifically, 7.1: observe and use evidence-based risk assessment tools to determine need for support and intervention to optimise mobility and safety, and to identify and manage risk of falls using best practice risk assessment approaches; 7.2: use a range of contemporary moving and handling techniques and mobility aids; 7.3: use appropriate moving and handling equipment to support people with impaired mobility; and 7.4: use appropriate safety techniques and devices.

Expected knowledge

- Anatomy and physiology of the musculoskeletal system
- Principles of ergonomics/biomechanics
- Local policy on moving and handling.

Introduction

The ability to move easily and purposely is an essential part of living; unrestricted mobility is vital for independence and self-protection. Most patients will have some degree of immobility whether it is due to temporary causes, e.g. local anaesthesia, or more permanent ones, e.g. amputation or stroke. There are various medical conditions such as osteoporosis, rheumatoid arthritis and social conditions (e.g. morbid obesity) that affect independent mobility. Patients who are immobilised become vulnerable and dependent.

Content

Risk assessment	Moving and handling procedures for patients who are weight-bearing	Moving and handling procedures for patients who are unstable on feet or unable to bear weight
Devices and aids used in moving and handling		

Learning outcomes

- Demonstrate theory and application for the requirements and processes of risk assessment
- Explain safe core moving and handling manoeuvres
- Select the most appropriate device to manually handle a patient
- Correctly use the equipment for the manual handling of a patient.

Key background

Moving and handling patients is an intricate part of their care package. Many, due to their illness, will have compromised and limited mobility whether temporary or permanent. If not purposely thought through and actioned, poor moving and handling practices can cause serious injury to both staff and patients.

The principles of safe patient moving and handling should always be applied in the care management of all patients using adequately trained staff and additional devices and aids, for example slide sheets or hoists. Health and safety standards should be adhered to as dictated by the Health and Safety at Work Act 1974.

Manual handling procedures not only have inherent potential risks for injuries to nurses but can also compromise the patient's autonomy, dignity, comfort and safety. Thus, purposeful holistic patient assessment, risk assessment and meticulous care planning are paramount (focussing on the implementation of safe techniques can improve practices and ensure safety as far as possible).

Moving and handling guidelines (national and local) exist. However there is a lack of implementation and role-modelling of such guidance in clinical practice (Ramonaledi, 2017). All staff undertaking the practice of moving and handling should undergo training (and updates) so that they are competent in this skill and safe to both the patients and themselves.

RISK ASSESSMENT

Risk assessment involves a careful examination of what might cause harm, injury or illness to any individual. In moving and handling practice risk assessment will help the nurse to make informed clinical decisions and provide reasons for the interventions to be undertaken. A risk assessment should be performed at least within 24 hours of admission (including transfer from another area).

Generic Risk Assessment

Avoid wherever 'reasonable practical' hazardous manual handling activities should be avoided (MHOR1998).

Assess when avoiding such activities is challenging 'a suitable and sufficient assessment 'of potential hazards should be done to reduce the risks for harm or injury.

Reduce safe system of work and strategies to reduce the risks of injury should be put in place like educating the staff and providing appropriate equipment like hoists.

Review the risk assessment must be reviewed regularly to ensure the strategies to prevent injury remain effective and relevant.

Education – Staff must be suitably trained, follow appropriate systems of work and use equipment provided correctly.

Individual Risk Assessment - should include the abilities of the service user: Is it clinically safe to move the patient? What they can/cannot do independently.

Ability to support their own weight, any influencing factors such as pain, spasm, fatigue.

Participate in transferring.

Assistance with repositioning/sitting up.

Type of equipment required e.g. hoist, sling.

Arrangements for reducing the risk and dealing with falls.

The assessment should be performed by someone suitably trained and competent.

Assessment and planned interventions should be recorded on the patient's care plan.

An ongoing assessment with periodic review should also be factored into the care plan.

Types of risk assessment include:
1. Generic – type and frequency of moving and handling tasks. Equipment needed, staffing available, environment. Emergency procedural requirements such as fire evacuation.
2. Individual assessments – part of a care planning package to determine the moving & handling needs of a service user.

FIGURE 3.1 Risk assessment

SAFER PERSON PRACTICE FRAMEWORK
(BROOKS AND ORCHARDS, 2011)

Preparations by the nurse:
- *Identify* the rationale for procedure.
- *Refer* to patient's risk assessment documents. Assess their cognitive, emotional, physical capabilities, usual assistance, equipment and number of nurses required.
- *Make* decisions/judgements of appropriate handling interventions needed.
- *Undertake* a personal risk assessment identifying potential injury risks for all.
- *Seek* advice from others if needed.
- *Consider* safeguarding issues and cultural preferences for the patient during procedure.
- *Support* decisions (knowledge of professional guidelines and employers' policies).
- *Use* appropriate communication skills/attitudes to implement action plans in partnership with patients and colleagues.
- *Engage* staff with appropriate skills. A leader should coordinate procedure.
- *Ensure* team members are wearing suitable clothing and foot wear.
- *Consider* how to apply biomechanical principles to the context of current situation.

Preparation of patient
- Introduce self and obtain informed consent.
- Conduct a risk assessment (including patient's cognitive, emotional and physical capabilities.
- If applicable, the use of normal body movements should be encouraged first as these are natural and will facilitate autonomy.
- Teach, instruct and supervise patient to complete the movement independently where possible. If the patient is unable to the equipment should be introduced.
- Continuously provide information to patient and give reassurance.
- Give positive praise and encouragement, promoting comfort and dignity.
- Make patient comfortable.
- Document procedure.

Preparation of the environment and equipment:

- *De-cluttering or clearing* any obstructing furniture and dangers. Ensuring the environment is warm, well lit, clean and spacious.
- Floor surfaces should be safe (equipment use).
- Check handling equipment (safety).

FIGURE 3.2 Safer person practice framework

ELECTRIC PROFILING BED AND EQUIPMENT

Some patients rely on nurses partially or completely, to be safely moved and repositioned whilst in bed. There is a need to ensure their comfort and good skin integrity.

In addition to the standard hydraulic bed, there are currently different brands of electric profiling beds used in practice settings as part of ergonomic equipment provision (HSE, 2011). Thus minimising and avoiding risks associated with handling procedures. Patients can be sat up supported with pillows. The knee-break position can prevent patients slipping down the bed, while strong and steady bed sides can be used by semi dependent patients, to roll on to their side, with minimal help.

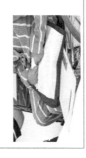

Transfer boards are steady solid plastic/wooden devices. Maximum working load is 130kg (20 stones). It is used to bridge gaps between two surfaces, e.g. bed to chair or chair to chair. Its use can help promote patient independence for seated transfers and provides a low friction glide between the two surfaces. For this to be used safely, the patient should have a good balance, able to sit and with good upper body strength.

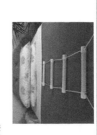

Rope ladders can promote independence to those in bed. They are simple devices that enable the patients to pull themselves up to a sitting position but with upper body strength and stability in order to do this.

Rope ladders are attached to the bottom part of the bedstead (stable part). This is performed by a physiotherapist. Check to ensure that it is secure, by pulling on it before the patient uses it.

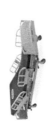

FIGURE 3.3 Electric profiling bed and equipment

SLIDE SHEETS

These are efficient low friction (avoiding skin damage) devices that are safe and easy to use. They are used in the transfer to beds, floors and chairs. Slide sheets can also be used to move patients up or down, turn to their sides in beds and transfer laterally and slide from tight awkward spaces when fallen. Slide sheets can be used independently for the patient to move themselves in bed. They can be disposable or reusable.

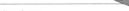

Types of sliding sheets:
> Roller sheets – tubular with open lateral sides. Some are padded. Rolling the top layer close to the patient and allow it to slide on the bottom layer.
> Lateral transfer slide sheets with/out extensions loops.

1. **Inserting Slide Sheet** – Bed brakes on. Adjust height of the bed to nurses' waists/pelvic crest.
2. Turn patient to the taller nurse and pull the patient over their body with comfortable levers.
3. Instruct/assist the patient to adopt a modified recovery position and turn their head in the direction of the turn.
4. Place patient's arm (side of turn) palm up on the pillow (protect the face). The far leg knee should be bent. If unable, use a small slide sheet to bend the knee.
5. Both nurses adopt a walking stance for stability.
6. The nurse towards the turn places arms across the patient's body and hands on shoulder and hip.
7. The other nurse superimposes their hands
8. Inform patient that on the command of 'Ready, Steady, Turn' they will be turned to an appropriate side.
9. On the command the nurse towards the turn gently pulls the patient towards self while the other gently nudges away from self. Slowly and smoothly.
10. The nurses maintain their natural postures by transferring their body weights to the back leg for the one pulling and the front leg for the one nudging.
11. Continue to hold patient on their shoulder and hip appropriately and adopt feet wide position for stability. The bed safety side can be pulled up.
12. Fold clean, appropriate body width and length, slide sheets into a longitudinal half and place parallel to the back of the patient. Place sheets from head to below the ankles of the patient.
13. The top half fold is folded as quarters towards the patient back (allowing easy retrieval).
14. Instruct the patient to roll on their back before being turned to the other side.
15. Pull and straighten sheets. Encourage & support patient to roll onto their back (middle of the slide sheets). Move patient up the bed.
16. Make the patient comfortable and remove the slide sheet.

1. **Removal of Slide Sheet** – After positioning the patient, examine the slide sheets to decide which side has the greatest amount of material showing.
2. Remove slide sheets from the side with most material.
3. Use natural hollow areas below the ankles, knees and under the neck (avoid the lumbar area as it is where most of the body weight is situated) to lunge and gently push an arm between the two sheets or layers of a tubular sheet.
4. The nurse on the opposite side should feed the corners of the pair of sheets in hand of the nurse removing them. Alternatively, the nurse removing the sheet grabs the bottom layer of the tubular sheet.
5. The nurse pulling out the slide sheet should place a free hand on the patient's knee area to support them and avoid change in position. Gently scoop/diagonally pull the sheets towards the patient's waist. Stop when resistance is encountered (preventing patient sliding).
6. Repeat procedure from under the patient's neck supporting the chest area, scoops and pulls the sheet, stopping at the waist.
7. Gently ease (from side to side) the slide sheets under the patient's waist.
8. Position patient comfortably and safety.

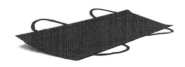

FIGURE 3.4 Slide sheets

STAND AID

Whilst some patients have difficulties walking, they may still be able to stand and hold their body weight confidently. Stand aids can be used to facilitate transfers from one seated position to another and help patients continue their rehabilitation towards independence. Some equipment has a turntable (for patient to stand on) that can be rotated 360 degrees. Shin pads can be used to provide protection and support for the patient's legs. It is height adjustable and has a foot pedal break (securing the turntable when patient is standing on it). To prevent risk of falling backwards, if the patient cannot stand independently for a short time will need the support of a nurse.

TWO nurses are required – one to support patient, the other to operate the equipment. Both should be trained and competent to use the equipment.

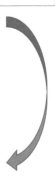

Procedure
1. Patient should be sitting on a chair or bed.
2. Patient should move their buttocks forward to front of chair/near edge of bed. Feet should be wide apart.
3. The nurse operating, should swivel the stand to the space between the patient's feet.
4. Patient's feet should be placed on the stand's footprints/non-slip squares. If it is if too painful or swollen for the patient to lift their feet, the supporting nurse should move them with slide sheets.
5. The operating nurse firmly holds the nearest handling bars firmly gaining a good base of support, places the front foot on the pedal brake, stabilising it.
6. The patient should place one hand on the arm of the chair/mattress (pushing up) and the other on the nearest handling bar of the stand (pulling up).
7. The supporting nurse helps the patient to stand.
8. Once patient is standing on the stand, the operating nurse takes off the brake and gently swivels 90 degrees.
9. The supporting nurse takes a wheelchair or patient ensuring that they can feel it behind their legs.
10. Put back on the brakes for the stand and the wheelchair.
11. Instruct patient to put hands on either arm rests of the wheelchair or on the mattress and slowly sit down.
12. Lift or slide feet off the turntable. Rotate the stand away, put foot plates of wheelchair in place. Put patient's feet on them.
13. Ensure patient is comfortable.

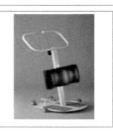

FIGURE 3.5 Stand aid

HOISTS

Hoists are one of the most common equipment used in moving and handling of people. Hoists, in order to avoid hazardous manual handling activities (to staff and service users) staff have to undergo relevant trining and use equipment as instructed by manufacturers guidance.

Hoists can be electric or battery operated. The three main types of hoists are:–

➢ *Fixed* – mounted on walls or floors and are convenient where space is lacking (e.g. bathrooms).

➢ *Overhead* – practical where space is limited and also promotes user independence. Due to their operational they promote safe carer postures (less back strain).

➢ *Mobile (passive or active)* – in diferent sizes and safe working loads capacities. Active hoists can be used in the rehabilitation and facilitation of patients with weight bearing capacity and balance, (stnading or relearning to walk). Passive hoists lift full body weights of dependent and fallen patients and are operated by the nurse. Common in practice settings.

Applying a sling
1. Patient to roll/assist patient onto their back
2. Roll the patient to a side
3. Fold sling in half (labels and handles on the outside)
4. Position along the back of the patient (from coccyx). If there is a head support, align the neck seam to the base of the neck.
5. Fold top half into a quarter and fold in the clips for patient comfort.
6. Roll patient on back, then the other side (for other nurse to access sling).
7. Unroll rest of sling and adjust for comfort.
8. Push hoist nearer to be visible to the patient from front. Lower to desirable height and attach the sling and hoist the patient.
9. Communicate and reassure patient all times whilst observing for signs of discomfort/anxiety.

Types of slings available:

➢ Divided leg sling – most common.
➢ Hammock style for those needing more support.
➢ Access sling – used for toileting and dressing.

Some slings are disposable but most are able to be washed at high temperatures and reused. Worn, split or torn slings should be immediately discarded. Also fabric that is fraying at the connection points, loose stitching or fabric weakness.

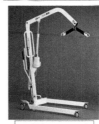

Mobile battery-operated hoist (picture in main book)

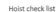

Hoist check list

- Staff using the hoist should be suitably trained and use in accordance to operating instructions.
- Conduct a manual handling risk assessment.
- Check the suitability of the hoist to safely carry the patient's weight and their needs. Check weight limit (at bottom of device).
- Check the maintenance date (normally every six months).
- Fully functional with no faults (including correct sling). Use with a full battery.
- Note the position of the emergency lowering device.
- Ensure the legs can be manipulated to open or close and that the spreader bar is in good condition.
- NEVER leave patient unattended. Or positioned where they could fall.

FIGURE 3.6 Hoists

ASSISTING AMBULANT PATIENTS

Adults and children who are ambulant are able to stand up. They have good upper body strength and control and are able to sit balanced and upright. They also have weight bearing capacities. They are able to move and position their buttocks to the front part of a chair or towards the edge of a mattress and push up to stand with hands on the armrests of the chair/mattress on the bed.

Despite this, some patients may or may not walk, depending on their physical conditions (ill health, pain), psychological and mental state (confused, anxious, fear, loss of confidence, mental health issues, depression) and will therefore need assistance and encouragement to do so. Do not force patients who are unwell with symptoms e.g. dizziness to stand/transfer.

Procedure – patient sitting upright in chair

1. Patient should put their hands on arm rests of chair, sit upright, lean forward with head up and facing forward.
2. Their buttocks should move towards the front (until middle of chair).
3. Position their feet hip width wide firm and flat on floor and under knees. Strong foot slightly back (helps push up when standing up). Head up and looking ahead.
4. Lone nurse adopts a lunge position on the side close to patient, looking forward.
5. Support patient with one hand on their front shoulder and the other on the lower back/hip furthest away.
6. Both nurse and patient gently rock back and forth on the command – 'Ready, Steady, Stand'. On stand, the patient pushes the hands off the arm rests and uses the strong foot to propel upwards and stands.
7. Nurse stands closer to patient on the weaker side/two nurses on either side. Nurses stabilise by transferring body weight with the back leg brought forward and the front one to step forward.
8. When patient is up and steady, the nurse(s) offer palm to palm hold or the back of a clenched fist for the patient's hand support (avoiding risk of injury to nurses' thumbs if gripped firmly by patient especially during a fall.
9. Allow patient to stand calmly for a while, feel stable & ready to start the walk.
10. Ask patient if they are ready to walk and clearly instruct to 'walk'. Steadily catch up with his or her pace to avoid pushing him or her.

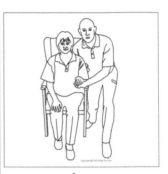

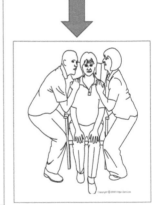

FIGURE 3.7 Assisting ambulant patients

WALKING WITH AIDS

Safety checks

➢ For the right height, there should be a slight flexion in the patients elbows. They should also be able to adequately straighten them to support patient's body weight when placed in front.
➢ The ferrules (rubber leg covering) should be intact.
➢ Undamaged handgrips.
➢ A firm and steady frame for single patient use.

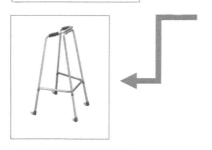

Walking (Zimmer) frame

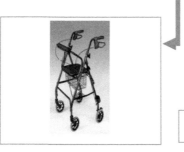

Frame with wheels

Procedure

1. Before standing the patient, place the frame by the patient's side (not too close to block forward movement) during transfer of body weight or too close in front of the patient as they may rush to hold on it.
2. Stand patient up and place the frame in front of them and at a safe distance. Both their hands should be placed on the handgrips.
3. Stands on the side and slightly behind the patient.
4. Patient should walk equal steps one at a time, towards the frame. If frame is too close, instruct the patient to put the frame a step In front, before stepping forward towards it.
5. Patient can lean slightly on the frame and take their body weight through the arms and walk equal steps (one at a time), to be in line with the back legs of the frame or at the centre of the frame.
6. Encourage the patient throughout the walk, to continue this pattern until he or she reaches a chair at the destination.
7. To sit, the patient should walk parallel and close to the seat of the chair.
8. After reaching the level of the furthest armrest of the chair (this will help bring the patient close to the chair and avoid walking backwards), turn frame slowly positioning it in front of the patient.
9. When patient feels chair behind their legs, they should reach for both the rests of the chair, ONE hand at a time and bend the knees and move backwards to sit.
10. Frames are specialised to meet the patient's needs (adult/child) e.g. with wheels/brakes/seats. These walking frames may also have wheels with brakes on the four legs.

FIGURE 3.8 Walking aids

Now test yourself: activity

1. What are the five components of a generic risk assessment?

2. Name three different types of hoists.

3. Which of the following statements are **true**?

   a) Ambulant patients have the ability to stand.

   b) Ambulant patients can sit but may veer to one side.

   c) Ambulant patients are able to move their buttocks towards the front of the chair.

   d) Ambulant patients have good lower body strength only.

4. **True** or **false**? A person using a walking aid should have slight flexion in their elbow.

5. Complete the following sentence:
   Slide sheets are ____ friction devices that are safe and ____ to use. They can be used to move the patient up or ____ the bed and ____ them from bed to chair. They are very ____ in health care settings.

Answers

1. **Avoid** hazardous manual handling activities.

    Assess for actual and potential hazards.

    Reduce the risks of injury by adopting a safe system of work.

    Review risk assessment regularly.

    Education of staff.

2. Fixed, overhead or mobile

3. a) and c) are true.

4. True.

5. Slide sheets are <u>low</u> friction devices that are safe and <u>easy</u> to use. They can be used to move the patient up or <u>down</u> the bed and <u>transfer</u> them from bed to chair. They are very <u>common</u> in health care settings.

Reflection: ask yourself

1. What do I know now that I didn't know before?

2. What am I confused/unclear about?

3. What areas do I need to focus on?

4. My action plan for further learning (make objectives SMART – Specific/Measurable/Achievable/Realistic/Time-bound):

CHAPTER 4

Therapeutic and procedural positions

Tina Moore

Overview

There are patients who will become unable to reposition themselves due to a variety of problems (e.g. unconsciousness, breathlessness, weakness) and therefore rely on assistance from nurses to place them in the correct position for their illness. This change may be temporary or permeant and the degree of semi-independence to total dependence will vary. It is critical to put the patient in the correct position in order to avoid the risk of injury and subsequent problems.

Link to *Future Nurse Proficiencies* (NMC 2018)

Platform 3 Assessing needs and planning care (Sections 3.5; 3.7).
Annexe B, Part 2: Procedures for the planning, provision and management of person-centred nursing care. Specifically, 3.3: use appropriate positioning and pressure-relieving techniques; 3.4: take appropriate action to ensure privacy and dignity at all times; and 3.5: take appropriate action to reduce or minimise pain or discomfort.
and
Use evidence based, best practice approaches for meeting needs for care and support with mobility and safety, accurately assessing the person's capacity for independence and self care and initiating appropriate intervention: specifically 7.1: observe and use evidence-based risk assessment tools to determine need for support and intervention to optimise mobility and safety, and to identify and manage risk of falls using best practice risk assessment approaches; 7.2: use a range of contemporary moving and handling techniques and mobility aids; 7.3: use appropriate moving and handling equipment to

support people with impaired mobility; and 7.4: use appropriate safety techniques and devices.

Expected knowledge

- Promotion of a healthy back and spine
- Principles of biomechanics
- Ergonomics – natural body movement
- Anatomy and physiology of the musculoskeletal system
- Local trust/hospital policies on moving and handling.

Introduction

Patient positioning activities are an essential part of the patient's care package. It is the duty of the nurse not to inflict any harm or injury to themselves, colleagues or indeed patients.

When possible, the position during surgery should be one that would be comfortable if the patient were fully awake. Patients should be questioned about limited range of motion and their ability to lie comfortably in the expected position. If questions arise, the patient should be placed in the anticipated position as a trial before sedation or induction of anaesthesia. Positioning can cause cardiovascular and respiratory issues with some patients.

Content

Principles of positioning the patient	Common positions used	Indications and benefits of these positions
Problems associated with certain positions	Benefits to the patient placed in certain positions	

Learning outcomes

- Demonstrate theory and practice of the principles of patient positioning
- Describe the common positions that patients may be required to adopt whilst in bed or a chair
- Identify the benefits of these positions for the patient
- Critically appraise the potential risks of such positions on the patient.

Key background

Not much guidance exists in relation to patient positioning; most of the literature on this topic relates to positioning patients during surgery. Lessons may be learnt from this sector. There are three identified elements of safe positioning, i.e. knowledge, planning and teamwork. Nurses should have knowledge about the principles of appropriate and safe patient positioning, eliminating risks to the patient, their colleagues and themselves at all times. They should also have knowledge and understanding of the complications that could arise, including injury and physiological changes within the patient.

The aims of positioning patients are to avoid and minimise complications such as pressure ulcers, breathing problems, effects of raised intracranial pressure; to maintain homeostasis; to protect anatomical structures and avoid injuries (such as nerves, digits, spine); and to ensure and promote patient comfort, privacy and dignity.

Positioning morbidly obese patients can pose multiple physiological challenges. The ideal positioning for such patients may not be possible; therefore, optimal positioning that provides as much comfort for the patient as possible whilst minimising risks should be achieved. The sheets that the patient is lying on should be wrinkle-free. The use of additional foam or gel positioning devices may actually contribute to the development of pressure ulcers due to the weight of the patient compressing the devices.

Those patients with diabetes and peripheral vascular disease (PVD) are also considered to be high-risk patients for complications. Both types of patients (but particularly those with PVD) may have pre-existing tissue ischemia. They may also have a history of hypertension, increasing their risk of hypotensive episodes on moving their position. Here, in order to prevent an abnormal reduction in blood pressure, patients should be moved gradually. Nicotine causes vasoconstriction resulting in decreased tissue oxygenation. Therefore, smokers are more susceptible to developing vasoconstriction of the cutaneous blood vessels. This is also the primary cause of PVD.

PATIENT POSITIONING

In order to prevent complications of immobility and injury the patients neural body alignment has to be maintained. In addition, preventing hyperextension of the neck and limbs and extreme lateral rotation in order to prevent injury. Quick, non-purposeful jerky movements of the patient should also be avoided.

In order to promote safe patient positioning there should be the following:

- Adequate number of staff (not just for preventing injury during moving and handling but to protect cannulas, tubes, catheters etc.) and adequate, appropriate fully functioning positioning devices are available.
- Knowledge of theoretical and practical of correct posture, alignment and pressure points. Preventing pressure ulcers, foot drop and contractures.
- Proper positioning is also vital for providing comfort for patients who are bedridden or have decreased mobility related to a medical condition or treatment. When positioning a patient in bed, supportive devices such as pillows, rolls, and blankets, along with repositioning, can aid in providing comfort and safety.

Risk of pressure ulcers
The patient's body should not in a position where there is a concentration on one area/pressure point in order to avoid pressure injuries. Pressure ulcers, localized injuries to skin or underlying tissue, can occur because of pressure or pressure in combination with shear and/or friction. Some patients may not be in a position to communicate feelings/warning signs of the consequences of too much pressure, e.g. numbness, tingling.

Contributing risk factors to the development of pressure ulcers can be either intrinsic factors or extrinsic factors. Intrinsic factors can include the overall health of the patient, and pre-existing conditions such as respiratory or circulatory disorders, diabetes mellitus, anaemia, malnutrition, advanced age, and body size.

Extrinsic factors may include Additional causes of pressure intensity (e.g. bedding) and length of time spent in that position. In addition, the musculoskeletal system of the patient may be subjected to stress during positioning. If the patient is receiving anaesthesia and muscle relaxants, these can depress pain, pressure receptors and muscle tone. Therefore, the normal defence mechanisms cannot guard against joint damage or muscle stretch and strain.

Guidance – Patient Positioning

- Explain procedure
- Obtain consent
- Maintain privacy and dignity
- Encourage patient to assist as much as possible
- Teach patient/provide instructions
- Get appropriate help
- Use correct and working devices
- Raise bed so that weight is at the level of the nurse's centre of gravity
- Frequent position change
- Avoid friction and shearing
- Good body mechanics:
  - ❖ Position self close to patient
  - ❖ Keep neck back and pelvis aligned
  - ❖ Flex knees and feet wide apart
  - ❖ Use arms and legs (not back)
  - ❖ Tighten abdominal and gluteal muscles in preparation for moving

FIGURE 4.1 Patient positioning

SUPINE POSITION

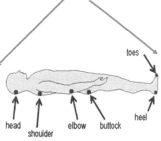

The **supine** or dorsal decubitus position is where the patient lays horizontally with their face and torso facing upwards. This position is used for surgical procedures such as head, neck abdominal, thoracic and cardiac. Post lumber puncture.

Not comfortable for long periods of time. The neck should be in a neutral position (with folded towel or pillow under head). Arms should always be maintained in a neutral thumb-up position. Legs, often positioned with knees slightly flexed resting on pillows (alleviates strain on lumbar spine).

Avoid in pregnancy (vena cava pressure & hypotension).

Supine position - pressure points

Being placed from an upright to supine position can cause the intra-abdominal contents and diaphragm to shift, compressing lung tissue causing a decrease in functional residual capacity and eventual atelectasis.

Increased venous return and pre load and eventual decrease in heart rate, stroke volume, and contractility.

Poor positioning can cause injury to the brachial plexus nerve (a combination of the C5-T1 nerve roots forming trunks, divisions, cords, and then branches to create the ulnar, radial, median, axillary and musculocutaneous nerves). Symptoms – weakness/ inability to move muscles/ lack of movement in arm, shoulder and hand.

At risk of multiple pressure ulcers.

PRONE POSITION

The **prone** (ventral decubitus) position is where the patient lays face down with their legs extended. position. It is not used frequently in general care areas (mainly in critical care).

The advantage is that it can improve oxygenation in patients with adult respiratory distress syndrome (ARDS) and decreasing mortality. improves the functional residual capacity of the lungs, reducing lung collapse and improving gaseous exchange. It also assists in moving secretions using gravity to assist in improving gaseous exchange and oxygenation.

Monitor for hypotension caused by pressure on vena cava. Shoulder dislocation and brachial plexus injury can occur when arms are placed above head. Move arms slowly in an arc position with elbows flexed, should not be extended >90°.

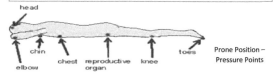

Prone Position – Pressure Points

It is important that the eyes, nose, ears, mouth do not have any pressure otherwise damage may occur.

Avoid too much pressure on other body parts such as toes, nose, ears, forehead, breast (female), shoulder, chest, genitalia (men), and pelvis as this can cause hypoperfusion, ischaemia and swelling. Ensure correct cushioning or those areas. Peripheral nerve compression injury can also occur.

Place pillows/wedges under shoulders and hips (helps allow chest expansion), pillow under feet and pillow/doughnut under head (helps with pressure relief.

FIGURE 4.2 Supine and prone

LATERAL POSITIONS

In the lateral position the patient lies on one side, either the right side (right lateral where patients right side is in contact with the bed) or left side (left lateral where their left side is in contact with the bed). It is important to maintain good spinal alignment, sufficient stabilisation of limbs and support of extremities (e.g. hands and feet) to prevent injury.

The top knee, and arm are flexed and supported by pillows (particularly in between the legs) for patient comfort. Increase in flexion of the top hip, knee and placing the upper leg in front of the body provides a wider gap achieving greater stability and balance.

Benefits of lateral positioning includes increased patient comfort and minimises /prevents the risk of complications from bed rest. This position helps take off pressure from the more common pressure points (particularly the coccyx), preventing pressure injury; and reduced deep vein thrombosis, pulmonary emboli, atelectasis, and pneumonia (by still maintaining adequate oxygen delivery and tissue oxygenation).

This is the position adopted when giving an enema or suppository. It is also common for colorectal, thoracic and hip surgery.

This position may not be appropriate for all patients, particularly those susceptible to cardiopulmonary and circulatory problems and instability.

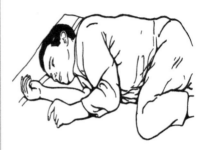

Risks

Whilst the lateral position relieves pressure on the sacrum and heels there are potential problems. These include:

➢ **Change in body weight distribution** – most of the body weight is distributed to the lateral aspect of the lower scapula, the lateral aspect of the ilium, and the greater trochanter of the femur, leading to:
➢ **Pressure to points on the dependent side of the body**, e.g. ears, shoulders, ribs, hips, knees and ankles, as well as brachial plexus injury, venous pooling, diminished lung capacity and DVT. A pressure-reducing or mattress or pillow/pressure relieving aids should be used as indicated.

FIGURE 4.3 Lateral positions

FOWLER POSITIONS

Known as 'standard' patient position. It is a sitting position where the top of the bed/chair is raised. Legs may be straight or flexed at the knees. The incline can range from 15–90 degrees depending on the variant of the fowlers position:

High Fowler – 60–90 degrees
Semi Fowler – 30–45 degrees
Low Fowler – 15–30 degrees

Generally, **high fowler** positions is used for patients with respiratory problems (with absence of cardiac contra indications) to facilitate better lung expansion and improve gaseous exchange. Also aids oral and nasogastric feeding. **Semi fowler** position is used for patients with breathing difficulties and/or cardiac problems. Passing of naso-gastric tube. **Low fowler** is used for patients with cardiac problems, head trauma, raised intra cranial pressure. Following surgery/procedures.

Risks – High fowlers position is uncomfortable for extended period. Patients with weak upper bodies may slump in the bed. There is also added pressure to the coccyx area.
Semi fowler position Is deemed the most comfortable.

There is an increased risk of skin injury (shearing/sliding in bed) and lower extremities DVT. Increased pressure risk to the scapulae, sacrum, coccyx, ischium, back of knees, and heels.

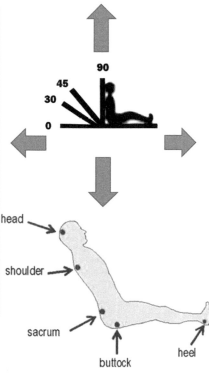

Pressure points

FIGURE 4.4 Fowler positions

ORTHOPNOEIC AND TRENDELENBURG POSITIONS

Orthopnoeic or **tripod position** is used for patients with breathing difficulties and who are dyspnoeic and breathless. The patient is sat in an upright, sitting position in bed, side of the bed or in a chair. The patient may get relief by having a bed table and pillows in front of them to lean and rest on.

This position facilitates respiratory expansion, makes it easier to breath, by facilitating the patients ability to use abdominal muscles and decrease diagrammatic pressure. It is also used during procedures such as thoracentesis and insertion of a chest drain.

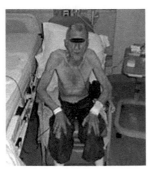

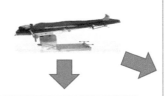

Trendelenburg position – patient is supine, the head/body tilted downwards approximately 15° and is lower than the feet.
This position can be used for pelvic, lower abdominal, colorectal and gynaecological surgeries. Insertion of central venous catheters.
It is also sometimes used in situations such as hypotension but there is currently no conclusive evidence to support this practice.
The modified Trendelenburg position is when the head is level with the body and legs are passively raised in the supine position.

Problems associated with the Trendelenburg position:

➢ Anxiety and restlessness
➢ Increased work of breathing and progressive dyspnoea
➢ Hypoventilation and atelectasis (reduced respiratory expansion)
➢ Altered ventilation/perfusion ratios from gravitation of blood to the poorly ventilated lung apices
➢ Increased intracranial pressure (increasing cranial venous congestion)
➢ Cephalad shift of abdominal contents causing pressure in the thoracic cavity (impairs venous return, leading to a further decreased cardiac output and hypotension)
➢ Increase risk of aspirating gastric contents
➢ Sliding and shearing of the skin

Trendelenburg position is usually not indicated in patients:

➢ who are hypotensive
➢ whose mechanical ventilation is difficult/has decreased vital capacity
➢ with increased intracranial pressure
➢ with cerebral oedema
➢ who have increased intraocular pressure
➢ with ischaemia of the lower limbs

FIGURE 4.5 Orthopnoeic and Trendelenburg

Activity: now test yourself

1. List four complications from positioning patients.

2. Which of the following statements are **true**?

   a) High Fowler position (60°–90°) is used for patients with cardiac disease having breathing problems.

   b) Semi Fowler position (30°–45°) is used for patients with both respiratory and cardiac problems.

   c) The best position to give a suppository or enema is the left lateral position.

   d) The orthopnoeic position is also described as the tripod position.

3. What is the 'modified Trendelenburg position'?

4. What are the intrinsic and extrinsic factors that contribute to pressure ulcers?

Answers

1. Any of the following:

    Pressure ulcers, uncomfortable, compression of vital organs (e.g. lung/heart), breathing difficulties, reduction of blood pressure, nerve injury, muscle weakness, sliding and shearing of skin, contractures, embolism formation leading to thrombosis.

2. b), c), and d) are true.

    a) is false. Cardiac problems are a contra indication of this position as the workload of the heart will be increased leading to further cardiac problems

3. The modified Trendelenburg position is when the head is level with the body and the legs are passively raised.

4. Intrinsic factors relate to the health of the patient. So, any current or past medical problems (e.g. respiratory or circulatory disorders, diabetes mellitus, PCD).

    Extrinsic factors are causes external to the patient (e.g. length of time spent in position, unequal distribution of weight when positioning).

Reflection: ask yourself

1. What do I know now that I didn't know before?

2. What am I confused/unclear about?

3. What areas do I need to focus on?

4. My action plan for further learning (make objectives SMART — Specific/Measurable/Achievable/Realistic/Time-bound):

CHAPTER 5

Legal aspects of moving and handling

Tina Moore

Overview

In care settings, manual handling operations commonly include the handling or moving of service users. Manual handling is a major contributor to yearly injuries sustained within the workplace. There are a number of legal frameworks and legislations to protect employees (and patients) from harm and injury.

Link to *Future Nurse Proficiencies* (NMC 2018)

Platform 1 Being an accountable professional (Sections 1.1; 1.2; 1.7; 1.8).

Platform 6 Improving safety and quality of care (Sections 6.1; 6.3; 6.5; 6.6).

Annexe B, Part 2: Procedures for the planning, provision and management of person-centred nursing care. Specifically, 3.3: use appropriate positioning and pressure-relieving techniques; 3.4: take appropriate action to ensure privacy and dignity at all times; and 3.5: take appropriate action to reduce or minimise pain or discomfort.

and

Use evidence based, best practice approaches for meeting needs for care and support with mobility and safety, accurately assessing the person's capacity for independence and self care and initiating appropriate intervention: specifically, 7.1: observe and use evidence-based risk assessment tools to determine need for support and intervention to optimise mobility and safety, and to identify and manage risk of falls using best practice risk assessment approaches; 7.2: use a range of contemporary moving and handling techniques and mobility aids; 7.3: use appropriate moving and handling equipment to support people with impaired mobility; and 7.4: use appropriate safety techniques and devices.

Expected knowledge

- Accountability and responsibility
- Basic understanding of the legal framework within the UK
- The Code (NMC, 2018)
- Trust policy on moving and handling practices.

Introduction

Accountability is an integral part of professional practice, requiring the nurse to give explanation and justification for actions and omissions in relation to care. Definitions of accountability reflect the expectation that justification should be evidence-based.

The term 'accountability' suggests that an approach to a situation has been systematic (assessed, planned and evaluated). Accountability assumes the nurse has the necessary knowledge, skill, experience and subsequent authority to carry out the plan.

Arenas of accountability include:

- *Patient*: Nurses are primarily accountable to the patients within their care; they have a legal and professional duty to act in the best interest of the patient (civil liability).
- *Professional body*: NMC – Professional Conduct Committee (professional liability).
- *Employers*: Nurses in breach of employment contract may face an industrial tribunal.
- *Public*: Nurses can be tried in the criminal law courts (criminal liability), if a crime is suspected of being committed.

Professional practice demands that the nurse be competent and have mastery in the chosen field of nursing. This mastery should also hold a genuine passion and vision for nursing, coupled with an endeavour towards excellence and quality. If a qualified nurse fails to follow The Code (NMC, 2018), they may be reported to the NMC for an investigation into their 'fitness to practice'.

Content

Legal aspects of moving and handling	Legislation (Health and Safety at Work Act 1974)	Regulations (LOWER/PUWER)
Employers responsibilities	Employees responsibilities	

Learning outcomes

- Demonstrate knowledge and understanding of laws and regulations relating to the work practice of moving and handling
- Critically analyse the impact of moving and handling practices on the nurse
- Discuss the employer's and employee's legal responsibilities in the workplace.

Key background

Negligence

The employer has a legal duty of care not to place the employee under undue and unnecessary risk of injury. If the court of law proves that the employer failed in this duty, there are usually consequences. If harm is suffered by staff or patients from the use of faulty equipment, poor moving and handling techniques, wrong use of equipment, the tort of negligence is applied. This tort is the most commonly used legal concept in maintaining standards. It is based on tort law, and refers to a civil wrong. Patients and staff have a range of rights that will be protected by the civil courts.

When an individual considers suing for damages for harm suffered, the burden of proof, according to the law, lies with that individual. This burden of proof depends on a balance of probabilities.

The law of negligence can be used in two different ways:

1. to sue another person for compensation, harm or damage
2. to indicate that behaviour has fallen below required standards.

To succeed in an action, the plaintiff must show:

1. that the existence of a duty to care was owed to them by the defendant
2. a breach of that duty by the defendant
3. that as a result the plaintiff has suffered damage (and the harm suffered must have been reasonably foreseeable).

Duty of care

A duty of care to someone in the law of negligence means being obliged to take his or her interest into account. Reasonable care must be taken to avoid acts or omissions that can reasonably be foreseen to cause injury/harm.

A duty of care is owed when:

- any person is voluntarily attended to by a nurse in an emergency situation, whether on or off duty (Kent v Griffiths, 2000)
- any patients present themselves in hospital and nurses have knowledge of that patient.

There is a contractual agreement between patient and nurse; therefore a legal duty of care is owed.

Breach of duty of care

As discussed, the employer has a duty of care to ensure that the equipment is safe to use and is well maintained, and that staff have the necessary training to enable safe moving and handling techniques. The staff have a duty of care to attend the training sessions offered by employers. A standard of care owed to the patient needs to be identified and examined. Patients depend upon nurses and their standards of professional conduct. The standard of care provided by any professional person must be of a higher level than that of a novice. The courts require an acceptable reasonable standard to be followed; a standard that would be supported by competent professional opinion and practice (Griffith and Dowie, 2019). The nurse is expected to exhibit the expertise normally demonstrated by a competent nurse, i.e. to comply with the Bolam Test (Bolam v Friern Barnet, 1957). The Bolam test states that the person executing the skill should be an ordinarily skilled person exercising and professing to have the skill (someone suitably qualified and experienced), be a reasonably competent practitioner, and be acting in accordance with acceptable practice at the time as proper (as defined by a reasonable body of professional opinion).

Courts rely on expert evidence to give an opinion of what is deemed to be a reasonable action and the accepted practice in a given situation. It is assumed that their opinions will be based on current evidence in order to provide a logical reason. Documentation for consultation in regarding acceptable standard of performance would be NMC documentation, policies, procedures and national/local guidelines.

The law would not find it acceptable to say that, in providing patient care, a nurse would be legally expected to perform at a lower standard of care. Some situations require deviation from the normal accepted procedures. Nurses can deviate from accepted standards, but need to clearly document why (Griffith and Dowie, 2019).

Causation

Causation seeks to examine the causal link between the failure of the defendant to follow the approved practice and the harm suffered by the patient which must have been reasonably foreseeable (Griffith and Dowie, 2019). There is a need to establish a causal link between the breach of duty to care by the nurse and the harm suffered by the patient.

LEGAL ASPECTS

Even though this is not a skill it is important to understand the legal aspects involved in a skill.

Laws protect all people's human rights, in social and work places. Employers and organisations use laws and institutional policies, as guidelines for acceptable standards of work practices, to ensure quality of services and safety for all.

It is imperative that nurses develop a sound knowledge of key laws and regulations, pertaining to moving and handling and understand their impact on practice.

Within moving and handling, Health and Safety Laws are designed to:

> ➤ help to reduce and avoid risks of injuries, to patients, nurses and their colleagues during their work.
> ➤ set guidance and duties for both employers and employees, to ensure safe workplaces and practices.
> ➤ describe safe standards of work, risk assessment processes and the appropriate use of suitable equipment for good handling practice.
> ➤ Application these laws in practice are supported by NMC (2018) and Employers' policies.

The Acts, Regulations and Policies relevant to moving and handling practice are:
- The Health & Safety at Work Act (HASWA or HASAWA) 1974
- Manual Handling Operations Regulations 1998 (MHOR)
- Reporting of Injuries, Diseases and Dangerous Occurrences Regulation 1995 (RIDDOR)
- Management of Health & Safety at Work Regulations 1999
- Provision & Use of Work Equipment Regulations 1998 (PUWER)
- Lifting Operations and Lifting Equipment Regulations 1998 (LOLER)
- Human Rights Act 1998
- Disability Discrimination Act 1995
- Mental Capacity Act 2005
- NMC Professional Code of Conduct 2018
- Trust policies

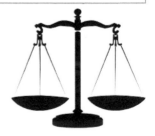

FIGURE 5.1 Legal aspects

HEALTH AND SAFTEY AT WORK ACT 1974

The aim of the Act is to ensure 'health, safety and welfare of people at work, and to protect people, other than those at work against risks to their health and safety arising out of work activities...'. The onus is on the employer to uphold safe work places, 'so far as is reasonably practicable'. Meanwhile, employees are expected to collaborate and comply with the employer's policies and safe systems of the work to support safety initiatives (HSWA1974).

The employers' duties under HSWA 1974
➢ Ensure and maintain a safe and healthy work environment (both physically and psychologically).
➢ Provide training, supervision and information on safety.
➢ Provide and regularly maintain appropriate work equipment and protective clothing.
➢ Provide policies and set up safe systems work (including processes for reporting accidents).
➢ Avoid employees undertaking manual handling activities with high risks of injuries.
➢ Appoint a competent health and safety officer.

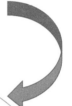

The employees' responsibilities under HSWA 1974
➢ Should attend training to ensure safe practice.
➢ Follow the employer's policies and safe systems of work.
➢ Use provided equipment appropriately and report any malfunctions.
➢ Report any ill health which could be made worse by work activities.
➢ Ensure personal health and safety and that of others who could be affected by their actions or omissions (including risk assessments).

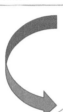

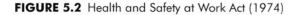

All staff should have knowledge and understanding of local health & safety policies.
All staff should attend mandatory basic training on moving and handling.
All staff using equipment to aid moving and handling should undergo structured and appropriate training. This should be competency based and assessed as such.
Correct number of staff should handle the equipment. Normally one to operate the equipment safely and the other observing the patient for signs of discomfort or potential hazards.
All equipment should be maintained to the highest standards and serviced frequently.

FIGURE 5.2 Health and Safety at Work Act (1974)

MANUAL HANDLING OPERATIONS
REGULATIONS 1992 (AMENDED 2002)

The Moving and Handling Operation Regulation 1998 (MHOR) (amended 2002 aim is to reduce the incidence and prevalence of musculoskeletal disorders (MSDs) arising from the manual handling of loads at work. These regulations also highlight the duty of the employer to engage in risk assessment in the work place to prevent and reduce potential injuries from manual handling activities 'as far as reasonably practical'.

Responsibilities of the employer

➤ Avoid hazardous manual handling so far as is reasonably practicable. Could redesign the task to avoid moving the load or by automating or mechanising the process.

➤ Make a suitable and sufficient assessment of any hazardous manual handling operations that cannot be avoided.

➤ Reduce the risk of injury from those operations so far as is reasonably practicable. Where possible providing mechanical assistance like hoists. Where this is not reasonably practicable, to explore ways of changing the task, the load and working environment.

Responsibilities of an employee

➤ Employees have the duty to follow the employer's safe system of work in place to promote safety for all.

➤ Employees' activities should not endanger, harm or put others safety at risk.

➤ Use provided equipment fully and properly.

➤ Co-operate with the employer on all health and safety issues and plans in place including wearing suitable clothing and footwear.

➤ Inform the employer if they identify hazardous handling activities.

Risk Assessment (HSE, 2004)

❖ **Avoid** – wherever 'reasonable practical' hazardous manual handling activities should be avoided (MHOR, 1998).

❖ **Assess** – when avoiding such activities is challenging 'a suitable and sufficient assessment' of potential hazards should be done to reduce the risks for harm or injury.

❖ **Reduce** – safe system of work and strategies to reduce the risks of injury should be put in place like educating the staff and providing appropriate equipment like hoists.

❖ **Review** – the risk assessment must be reviewed regularly to ensure the strategies to prevent injury remain effective and relevant.

FIGURE 5.3 Manual Handling Operations Regulations (2002)

PROVISION AND USE OF WORK EQUIPMENT REGULATION (PUWER) (1998)

These regulations provide guidance in relation to all equipment and machinery used in the workplace not mentioned by LOLER. The PUWER Regulations aim to make working life safer for everyone using and coming into contact with equipment: employers and employees, contractors, suppliers, and others. Like all regulations, they need to be studied closely. The words have been chosen carefully and sometimes have a precise legal meaning. At other times, you need to interpret the Regulations according to your own situation.

Duties of the employer under PUWER 1998 to ensure that equipment provided is:

➢ Suitable for use and for the purpose and conditions under which is used.
➢ Maintained in safe condition for use so that people's health and safety is not at risk e.g. cleaned.
➢ Inspected in certain circumstances to ensure it is and continues to be safe for use, this could be a competent employee e.g. visual inspection and checking functions before use.
➢ Ensure risks are eliminated by following software measures e.g. follow safe systems of work and provide adequate information and training.
➢ Ensure people using the equipment receive adequate training and information.

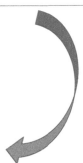

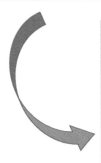

Risk assessments
Risk assessments are necessary due to the legal obligations of protecting yourself and your employees when using equipment and/or machinery. The risk assessments include:

➢ Recognising potential hazards and making a record of them
➢ Considering the possible harm caused by any outcomes of a risk assessment in order to identify the necessary actions to lessen or eradicate these risks
➢ Identifying an alternative way of doing things in order to reduce or eliminate risks

FIGURE 5.4 Provision and Use of Work Equipment Regulation (PUWER) (1998)

THE LIFTING OPERATIONS AND LIFTING EQUIPMENT REGULATION (LOLER) 1998

LOLER promotes safe use of equipment for moving and handling, in work environments. This regulation covers lifting and lowering equipment such as beds, hoists and slings (including attachments used for anchoring, fixing or supporting) used at work and private homes as part of work.

Duties of the employer under LOLER 1998
➢ Equipment provided should be strong, stable and suitable for intended purpose and environment.
➢ They must be installed or stored to prevent the risk of injury e.g. from equipment failing or load falling or striking people.
➢ Equipment must be marked visibly with information to be taken into account for its safe use e.g. Safe working load (SWL), slings.
➢ Equipment for lifting and lowering are examined and inspected six-monthly by a competent person who writes a report (and recommendations for appropriate actions if indicated) for the employer.
➢ All lifting operations are planned, supervised and carried safely by a competent person.

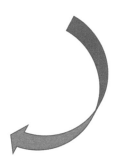

Where you undertake lifting operations involving lifting equipment you must:
- plan them properly
- using people who are sufficiently competent
- supervise them appropriately
- ensure that they are carried out in a safe manner

FIGURE 5.5 The Lifting Operations and Lifting Equipment Regulation (LOLER) (1998)

Activity: now test yourself

1. What are the consequences of employers/employees failing to conduct a risk assessment and the patient thus suffering harm?

2. What is the main purpose of health and safety laws?

3. **True** or **False**:

   'LOLER promotes safe use of equipment for moving and handling, in work environments. PUWER Regulations do not deal with equipment but instead concentrates on the knowledge, understanding and skill of staff in relation to moving and handling'.

4. List four main areas within the Health and Safety at Work Act (1974).

Answers

1. Consequences would involve issues around accountability and the Tort of Negligence, and prove in relation to: Duty of Care/Breach of Duty and Causation.

2. The main purposes of health and safety laws (supported by NMC 2018):

   - *help to reduce and avoid risks of injuries within the workplace*

   - *ensure safe workplaces and practices by setting standards and guidance*

   - *provide guidance on risk assessment processes and the appropriate use of suitable equipment.*

3. *False.* Both relate to the use of equipment within the workplace.

4. Any of the following:

   - *staff knowledge and understanding of local health and safety policies*

   - *that staff have attended mandatory basic training on moving and handling*

   - *appropriate staff training for moving/handling techniques and use of equipment*

   - *that staff have the correct number of competent colleagues involved in moving and handling patients*

   - *that all equipment used should be safe and fully functional.*

Reflection: ask yourself

1. What do I know now that I didn't know before?

```



```

2. What am I confused/unclear about?

```



```

3. What areas do I need to focus on?

```



```

4. My action plan for further learning (make objectives SMART – Specific/Measurable/Achievable/Realistic/Time-bound):

```



```

Bibliography

American College of Rheumatology (2015) Timed Up and GO (TUG). American College of Rheumatology. [online]: https://www.rheumato logy.org/I-Am-A/Rheumatologist/Research/Clinician-Researchers/ Timed-Up-Go-TUG. Accessed 20.05.20.

Bolam V Friern Barnet HMC (1957) All ER 118.

Brooks, A. and Orchard, S. (2011) Core Person Handling Skills. In: J. Smith (ed.), *The Guide to Handling of People*, 6th edn. Middlesex: Backcare.

Cummings, J. (2017) Blog: Valuing Patients Time. [online]: https://www. england.nhs.uk/blog/valuing-patients-time/. Accessed 01.04.20.

Department of Health (DH) (2019) The NHS Long Term Plan. [online]: https://www.longtermplan.nhs.uk/wp-content/uploads/2019/01/nhs-long-term-plan-june-2019.pdf. Accessed 20.05.2020.

Escape (2020) Enabling Self-Management and Coping with Arthritic Pain Using Exercise. [online]: https://escape-pain.org/. Accessed 20. 05.20.

Griffith, R. and Dowie, I. (2019) *Dimond's Legal Aspects of Nursing: A Definitive Guide to Law for Nurses*, 8th edn. Harlow: Pearson's Education Ltd.

Health and Safety Executive (HSE) (1974) Health and Safety at Work Act. [online]: https://www.hse.gov.uk/legislation/hswa.htm. Accessed 14.05.20.

Health and Safety Executive (HSE) (1998) Lifting Operations and Lifting Equipment Regulations (LOLER).

Health and Safety Executive (HSE) (2002) The Manual Handling Operations Regulations (as amended).

Health and Safety Executive (HSE) (2004) Manual Handling: Manual Handling Operations Regulations (1992). *Guidance on Regulations*, 3rd edn. London.

Health and Safety Executive (HSE) (2008) PUWER 1998. [online]: https:// www.hse.gov.uk/pubns/priced/puwer.pdf. Accessed 14.05.20.

Health and Safety Executive (HSE) (2011) Electric Profiling Beds in Health Care. https://www.hse.gov.uk/healthservices/epb-health-care. pdf. Accessed 16.07.20.

Health and Safety Executive (HSE) (2011) Getting to Grips with Hoisting People. https://www.hse.gov.uk/pubns/hsis3.pdf. Accessed 14.05.20.

BIBLIOGRAPHY

Kent V Griffiths (no. 3) 2000 2 WLR 1158.

MSD Manual (MSD) (2020) Biology of the Musculoskeletal System. [online]: https://www.msdmanuals.com/home/bone,-joint,-and-muscle-disorders/biology-of-the-musculoskeletal-system/bones. Accessed 01.05.20.

National Health Service (NHS) (2019) How to Sit at Your Desk Correctly - Healthy Body. [online]: https://www.nhs.uk/live-well/healthy-body/how-to-sit-correctly/. Accessed 20.04.20.

National Institute for Health and Care Excellence (2019) Assessing for Falls: Clinical Knowledge Summary. [online]: https://cks.nice.org.uk/falls-risk-assessment#!scenarioRecommendation. Accessed 15.04.20.

Nursing and Midwifery Council (NMC) (2018) *Future Nurse Proficiencies*. London. [online]: https://www.nmc.org.uk/globalassets/sitedocuments/education-standards/future-nurse-proficiencies.pdf. Accessed 03.07.20.

Nursing and Midwifery Council (NMC) (2018) *The Code: Professional Standards of Practice and Behaviour*. London: NMC.

Office for National Statistics (2016) Sickness absence in the UK labour market: 2016. https://www.ons.gov.uk/employmentandlabourmarket/peopleinwork/labourproductivity/articles/sicknessabsenceinthelabourmarket/2016. Accessed 20.05.20.

Office for National Statistics (2018) Sickness Absence in the UK Labour Market: 2018. [online]: https://www.ons.gov.uk/employmentandlabourmarket/peopleinwork/labourproductivity/articles/sicknessabsenceinthelabourmarket/2018. Accessed 20.05.20.

Public Health England and National Health Service (2019) Musculoskeletal Health: 5 Year Strategic Framework for Prevention across the Life Course. Crown Copyright. [online]: https://assets.publishing.service.gov.uk/government/uploads/system/uploads/attachment_data/file/810348/Musculoskeletal_Health_5_year_strategy.pdf. Accessed 20.05.20.

Ramonaledi, S. (2017) *Moving and Handling in: Moore T and Cunningham S (2017) Clinical Skills for Nursing Practice*. London: Routledge.

Royal College of Nursing (2019) Advice Guides: Moving and Handling. [online]: https://www.rcn.org.uk/get-help/rcn-advice/moving-and-handling. Accessed 16.07.20.

World Health Organization (2021) Musculoskeletal Conditions, Fact sheets. https://www.who.int/news-room/fact-sheets/detail/musculoskeletal-conditions. Accessed 12.02.21.

Yamato, T. P., Maher, C. G., Traeger, A. T., Wiliams, C. M., and Kampe, S. J. (2018) Do Schoolbags Cause Back Pain in Children and Adolescents? A Systematic Review. *British Journal of Sports Medicine*, 52: 1–6.

Index

Page numbers in *italics* denote figures.